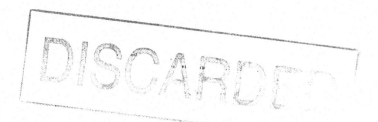
'This book is an essential read for any health professional working in the field of teenage and young adult cancer. It provides an exceptional combination of published evidence alongside personal and honest reflections of experts in this field. A range of thought-provoking case studies beautifully illustrate the complexity of supporting young people through their cancer journey and at last provides some practical advice for health professionals. Thank you for a much needed and wonderful book!'

Rachael Hough, *consultant haematologist, University College London Hospitals NHS Foundation Trust and professor of Haematology and Haematopoietic Stem Cell Transplantation, University College London*

'This comprehensive book traces the huge developments in the field of psych-oncology, identifying the apparent lack of psychological services for teenagers with cancer, and revealing the stigma around mental health in this area. Across its chapters, the book usefully describes the fundamental theoretical approaches, and differences therein, of psychotherapists, psychologists, and psychiatrists, to clarify the unique skills required when working in teenage and young adult psych-oncology. This includes a vivid survey of the challenges facing adolescents with cancer, exploration of the therapeutic relationship with young people who know they are dying, understanding trauma and the 'late effects' of childhood cancer, as well as the ways in which practitioners can support patients and their families to sustain hope in the midst of despair.'

Dorothy Judd, *child and adolescent psychotherapist and adult psychotherapist*

'This is an excellent and thought-provoking book which should be read widely by those interacting with adolescents and young adults with experience of cancer. Each chapter provides a holistic review of a particular area of psych-oncology which, using considered and diverse vignettes, professional reflections and evidenced based practice, brings to life the reality of adolescent and young adult cancer care. Clearly laid out and accessible this is a valuable first in addressing the important relationships between mind and body in the context of a key life stage with compassion and practicality.'

Louise Soanes, *chief nurse, Teenage Cancer Trust*

D1477727

PERSPECTIVES FROM A PSYCH-ONCOLOGY TEAM WORKING WITH TEENAGERS AND YOUNG ADULTS WITH CANCER

Exploring the work of a Psych-Oncology Team in an inpatient and outpatient setting, this powerful, interesting, and engaging book is about teenagers and young adults diagnosed with cancer.

As part of the few multidisciplinary teams of this type in the United Kingdom, the authors offer helpful insights into supporting young people and their families as they navigate this complex and devastating disease, writing on key areas such as trauma, the effects of early childhood cancer in adolescence and beyond, the social and cultural effects of cancer treatment, hope, and hopelessness, and questions of mortality. Each chapter contains a mixture of clinical reflections and patient vignettes, along with clear guidance about how to support patients and their families both during and after treatment, and at the point of death too.

With a compassionate approach to understanding the challenges for patients, their families, and clinicians alike, this is a book for nurses, doctors, occupational therapists, and physiotherapists, for parents and carers, and for young people who find themselves in this position and who can easily feel as though they are alone with their overwhelming feelings.

Jane Elfer is a child and adolescent psychotherapist. She worked at UCLH for 18 years, working in all paediatric departments but mainly in the paediatric cancer services. Prior to this, she had worked in CAMHS, social care, the NSPCC, and primary schools. Her professional doctorate looks at the emotional impact of adolescents donating bone marrow to a sibling. Since retiring from the NHS, she continues to work with children and young people, her professional body, and a charity for children in hospital.

Tavistock Clinic Series

Margot Waddell, Jocelyn Catty, & Kate Stratton (Series Editors)

Titles in the Tavistock Clinic Series include:

A for Adoption: An Exploration of the Adoption Experience for Families and Professionals, by Alison Roy

Assessment in Child Psychotherapy, edited by Margaret Rustin & Emanuela Quagliata

Childhood Depression: A Place for Psychotherapy, edited by Judith Trowell, with Gillian Miles

Child Psychoanalytic Psychotherapy in Primary Schools: Tavistock Approaches, edited by Katie Argent

Complex Trauma: The Tavistock Model, edited by Joanne Stubley & Linda Young

Conjunctions: Social Work, Psychoanalysis, and Society, by Andrew Cooper

Couple Dynamics: Psychoanalytic Perspectives in Work with the Individual, the Couple, and the Group, edited by Aleksandra Novakovic

Doing Things Differently: The Influence of Donald Meltzer on Psychoanalytic Theory and Practice, edited by Margaret Cohen & Alberto Hahn

Group Relations and Other Meditations: Psychoanalytic Explorations on the Uncertainties of Experiential Learning, by Carlos Sapochnik

Inside Lives: Psychoanalysis and the Growth of the Personality, by Margot Waddell

Internal Landscapes and Foreign Bodies: Eating Disorders and Other Pathologies, by Gianna Williams

Melanie Klein Revisited: Pioneer and Revolutionary in the Psychoanalysis of Young Children, by Susan Sherwin-White

Mourning and Metabolization: Close Readings in the Psychoanalytic Literature of Loss, by Rael Meyerowitz

New Discoveries in Child Psychotherapy: Findings from Qualitative Research, edited by Margaret Rustin & Michael Rustin

On Adolescence: Inside Stories, by Margot Waddell

Organization in the Mind: Psychoanalysis, Group Relations, and Organizational Consultancy, by David Armstrong, edited by Robert French

Psychoanalysis and Culture: A Kleinian Perspective, edited by David Bell

Researching the Unconscious: Principles of Psychoanalytic Method, by Michael Rustin

Sexuality and Gender Now: Moving Beyond Heteronormativity, edited by Leezah Hertzmann & Juliet Newbigin

Short-Term Psychoanalytic Psychotherapy for Adolescents with Depression: A Treatment Manual, edited by Jocelyn Catty

Surviving Space: Papers on Infant Observation, edited by Andrew Briggs

Sustaining Depth and Meaning in School Leadership: Keeping Your Head, edited by Emil Jackson & Andrea Berkeley

Talking Cure: Mind and Method of the Tavistock Clinic, edited by David Taylor

The Anorexic Mind, by Marilyn Lawrence

The Learning Relationship: Psychoanalytic Thinking in Education, by Biddy Youell

Therapeutic Care for Refugees: No Place Like Home, edited by Renos Papadopoulos

Therapeutic Interventions with Babies and Young Children in Care: Observation and Attention, by Jenifer Wakelyn

Thinking Space: Promoting Thinking about Race, Culture, and Diversity in Psychotherapy and Beyond, edited by Frank Lowe

Turning the Tide: A Psychoanalytic Approach to Mental Illness. The Work of the Fitzjohn's Unit, edited by Rael Meyerowitz & David Bell

Understanding Trauma: A Psychoanalytic Approach, edited by Caroline Garland

Waiting to Be Found: Papers on Children in Care, edited by Andrew Briggs

"What Can the Matter Be?": Therapeutic Interventions with Parents, Infants, and Young Children, edited by Louise Emanuel & Elizabeth Bradley

Young Child Observation: A Development in the Theory and Method of Infant Observation, edited by Simonetta M. G. Adamo & Margaret Rustin

PERSPECTIVES FROM A PSYCH-ONCOLOGY TEAM WORKING WITH TEENAGERS AND YOUNG ADULTS WITH CANCER

Thrown Off Course

Edited by
Jane Elfer

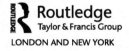

Routledge
Taylor & Francis Group
LONDON AND NEW YORK

Designed cover image: LEARNING TO THINK X, 2021, Blood on paper, 19.2 x 14.1 cm © Antony Gormley. Sir Antony Gormley shared the following description when he kindly provided permission to republish the image on the cover of this book: "a youth between sky and earth but rooted: vulnerable but alert, alive and looking out."

First published 2023
by Routledge
4 Park Square, Milton Park, Abingdon, Oxon OX14 4RN

and by Routledge
605 Third Avenue, New York, NY 10158

Routledge is an imprint of the Taylor & Francis Group, an informa business

© 2023 selection and editorial matter, Jane Elfer; individual chapters, the contributors; together with The Tavistock and Portman NHS Foundation Trust

British Library Cataloguing-in-Publication Data
A catalogue record for this book is available from the British Library

Library of Congress Cataloging-in-Publication Data
Names: Elfer, Jane, 1953– editor.
Title: Perspectives from a psych-oncology team working with teenagers and young adults with cancer : thrown off course / edited by Jane Elfer.
Description: Abingdon, Oxon ; New York, NY : Routledge, 2023. | Includes bibliographical references and index.
Identifiers: LCCN 2022038564 (print) | LCCN 2022038565 (ebook) | ISBN 9781032351353 (hardback) | ISBN 9781032351360 (paperback) | ISBN 9781003325475 (ebook)
Subjects: MESH: Neoplasms—psychology | Psycho-Oncology—methods | Cancer Survivors—psychology | Stress, Psychological—therapy | Terminal Care—psychology | Adolescent | Young Adult
Classification: LCC RC271.M4 (print) | LCC RC271.M4 (ebook) | NLM QZ 260 | DDC 616.99/40651—dc23/eng/20230125
LC record available at https://lccn.loc.gov/2022038564
LC ebook record available at https://lccn.loc.gov/2022038565

ISBN: 978-1-032-35135-3 (hbk)
ISBN: 978-1-032-35136-0 (pbk)
ISBN: 978-1-003-32547-5 (ebk)

DOI: 10.4324/9781003325475

Typeset in Palatino
by Apex CoVantage, LLC

This book is dedicated to all of the children, teenagers, young adults, and parents who have been treated at UCLH, regardless of whether or not they used our service

CONTENTS

SERIES EDITORS' PREFACE   xi

ABOUT THE EDITOR AND CONTRIBUTORS   xv

PREFACE   xvii

Introduction   1
    Jane Elfer

1   Overview: cancer in teenagers and young adults
    and psycho-oncology   7
    Mike Groszmann

2   The cancer journey   35
    Mike Groszmann

3   Adolescents with cancer: a journey interrupted   46
    Jane Elfer

4   Keeping young adults with cancer connected:
    a psychologist's reflections   62
    Anna Galloway

5   Cancer in adolescence from a trauma perspective   79
       Daniel Glazer

6   Reverberations through the mind:
       explorations of emotional complexities arising
       from childhood cancer and its "late effects"   93
       Petra A. M. Mohr

7   Hope and despair in the face of life-threatening disease   112
       Claudia Henry

8   Working with families where a young person
       is facing death   123
       James McParland, Cristian Pena, & Sara Portnoy

REFERENCES   145
INDEX   157

SERIES EDITORS' PREFACE

Since it was founded in 1920, the Tavistock Clinic—now the Tavistock and Portman NHS Foundation Trust—has developed a wide range of developmental approaches to mental health which have been strongly influenced by the ideas of psychoanalysis. It has also adopted systemic family therapy as a theoretical model and a clinical approach to family problems. The Tavistock is now one of the largest mental health training institutions in Britain. It teaches up to 600 students a year on postgraduate, doctoral, and qualifying courses in social work, systemic psychotherapy, psychology, psychiatry, nursing, and child, adolescent, and adult psychotherapy, along with 2,000 multidisciplinary clinicians, social workers, and teachers attending Continuing Professional Development courses and conferences on psychoanalytic observation, psychoanalytic thinking, and management and leadership in a range of clinical and community settings.

The Tavistock's philosophy aims at promoting therapeutic methods in mental health. Its work is based on the clinical expertise that is also the basis of its consultancy and research activities. The aim of this Series is to make available to the reading public the clinical, theoretical, and research work that is most influential at the Tavistock. The Series sets out new approaches in the understanding and treatment of psychological disturbance in children, adolescents, and adults, both as individuals and in families.

In *Perspectives from a Psych-Oncology Team Working with Teenagers and Young Adults with Cancer: Thrown Off Course*, edited by Jane Elfer, the authors describe their work with young people with cancer, or recovering from its longer-term effects. This psych-oncology team—more conventionally referred to as "psycho-oncology" but named in consultation with its young patients—comprises child psychotherapists, child psychiatrists, and psychologists. The contributions they each make to this book provide a wide range of perspectives on the extraordinary clinical work achieved in this unusual clinical centre, whose work, and its background, is expertly introduced by Mike Groszmann in chapter 1.

Teenagers' and young adults' voices and experiences are at the heart of this moving book. This is essential, for, as Elfer observes in her own chapter, introducing the subject of adolescents with cancer, young people keenly wish "not to be a patient but to be seen for who they are". Not only does she convey how hard a cancer diagnosis is for young people and their parents, she also draws attention to the challenges of accepting the offer of psychological or psychotherapeutic help: one father exclaims to his son: "Now you've gone mad, too?" This example, albeit extreme, helpfully paves the way for later vignettes in the book in which parents, or patients themselves, initially reject or avoid offers of support from the Psych-Oncology Team, which then have to be repeated, with both persistence and tact. Once these encounters have been negotiated, however, a sense of relationship emerges, articulated in Anna Galloway's chapter as a "co-creating": for instance, where she describes how a mother and daughter are supported by their therapist to co-create a way of living with the daughter's diagnosis of cancer.

Elfer's chapter, providing a grounding in adolescence and the particular impact of cancer at this time, also helps us to understand a recurring theme weaving throughout the book's vignettes: how often young people experience the very real impact of cancer on concrete aspects of their everyday lives—the ability to play football or to socialize, the loss of their hair—as catastrophic assaults on their emerging identity. These are among the small traumas that stand in for the profound ones. Daniel Glazer's chapter on trauma and growth picks this up too, in examples, for instance, of a girl hating the crutch that represents her weakness but also hating her friends' kindness in supporting her without it; and of a boy for whom a penalty kick becomes a matter of "life or death".

The team works not just in situations where the young people are going through cancer treatment, but also in those where the treatment had taken place years previously and they are dealing with its "late effects". As Petra Mohr writes, these effects can be felt particularly acutely in adolescence, the transitional time in which adulthood and independence beckon but the shadows of earlier traumas are keenly experienced and reworked.

One of her young adult patients worries that she has "bad genes" or is "damaged goods"; another protests against the metaphors of battle and recovery: "They say I survived, but I haven't. I died." As Claudia Henry attests in her chapter, it is common for young people to say, "My treatment is over, I should be happy, but I'm not, I feel so lost."

Perhaps Elfer and her authors are bravest where they confront the limitations of their work: where treatment fails, and the children or young people die. Facing this almost unbearable situation with both the patients themselves and, beforehand and afterwards, with their families, is an essential part of their work, and one that is highly valued. In the final chapter, James McParland, Cristian Pena, and Sara Portnoy discuss their feelings about working so closely with death in this way. The images they describe—from the father who needed to find a way to talk to his daughter about her sister's imminent death, to the parent who needed to think about their child's funeral even before the child died, to the mother who could only find a way to endure the memory of her lost child 18 months after her death—remain powerfully in the reader's mind. They are also difficult for the staff (the writers of these chapters, but also their clinician colleagues) to work with. How to avoid "burnout" and vicarious trauma is also attended to here, with Henry writing about a staff group focusing on processing the experiences, and about a theme of "gratitude and appreciation for life" that would reappear regularly as a response to working in this profoundly troubling but moving area. Anna Galloway writes of a teenage patient who died that "relationships were the sole reason for her to keep living", in particular "her ongoing connection to her father despite his death". She describes how she herself was helped after her patient's death by the experience of knowing and working with her, which remained with her. McParland, Pena, and Portnoy also describe the power of feeling, for families or professionals alike, that one is on shaky ground when confronted with death, and the need to find a "safe place to stand": a place that connects with one's sense of self, perhaps, or abilities, to provide a robust place from which to speak and connect.

One such place that emerges in the pages of this volume is the place for hope. Time and again, the authors turn, implicitly and explicitly, to hope: not just hope in medical treatment, but in the power of therapeutic conversations the writers are able to have with their young patients and their families, and the power of relationships. McParland, Pena, and Portnoy distinguish between false or defensive uses of hope and realistic or *reasonable* hope (borrowing from Kaethe Weingarten), emphasizing the use of "hope" as a verb: a collaborative endeavour. Henry recalls an Italian saying in her chapter: "Hope is the last thing to die." She links this to the Greek myth of Pandora's Box, which she weaves into her account of children and young people dealing with—she points out—not "post-traumatic stress" but actively being "in trauma" with cancer. She acknowledges the challenge posed for professionals by this dire situation, whereby to hope that their patients recover may be to "fail to be alongside them in their despair", yet "to acknowledge that they may die may mean we are not able to stay with the hope that they still need".

That hope may be seen as a collaborative endeavour is perhaps an apt metaphor for the work both of the team and of the book itself, rather fittingly represented in its final conversational chapter: a co-creation that movingly brings to a wider audience the work of the editor, the contributors, and their colleagues in this extraordinary clinical team.

ABOUT THE EDITOR AND CONTRIBUTORS

Anna Galloway is a clinical psychologist who has worked at a number of hospitals, including University College London Hospital (UCLH), the Royal Marsden, and Great Ormond Street Hospital. She is passionate about supporting those who are struggling with life-changing diagnoses. She also works in private practice with children, adolescents, and adults experiencing a variety of physical and mental health difficulties.

Daniel Glazer is a clinical psychologist and currently Clinical Lead for the child and adolescent psychology team at UCLH. He has worked since 2013 with young people with cancer, helping to shape and grow the Psych-Oncology Team at UCLH. Daniel is an active member of the UK teenage and young adult psycho-oncology network and has facilitated workshops and events for the Teenage Cancer Trust. Through his work, Daniel has developed a passion for narrative, existential, and trauma-informed therapies.

Mike Groszmann is a consultant child and adolescent psychiatrist and Clinical Lead for the Department of Child & Adolescent Psychological Medicine at UCLH. He has worked in psycho-oncology since 2012. He is Lead for Child & Adolescent Mental Health for UCL Medical School. His psychiatry training was at the Royal Free Hospital and then Tavistock and

Portman NHS Foundation Trust, where he also trained in systemic and psychodynamic psychotherapies.

Claudia Henry trained as a child and adolescent psychotherapist at the Tavistock and Portman NHS Foundation Trust after working as a hospital play specialist in a large paediatric hospital. Following qualification in 2006, she worked in a CAMHS service before joining the Psycho-Oncology Service, where she worked for six years. She currently works in a CAMHS service and on a Neonatal Intensive Care Unit in Surrey.

James McParland is a clinical psychologist working with people with health conditions and their families. He is interested in the power of narratives and the possibilities that emerge when we amplify the voices of those who join us in therapeutic dialogue.

Petra A. M. Mohr has worked at UCLH since 2015 as a child and adolescent psychotherapist in inpatient and outpatient clinics within the cancer and other paediatric services. Prior to this, she worked for more than twenty years within community centres, schools, play centres, and charities. Her doctorate, *Shut In and Cut Off?*, researched extreme social withdrawal—"Hikikomori"—focusing on young people who have shut themselves away inside their rooms.

Cristian Pena has specialized in working with adolescents and young adults throughout his career. Previously, he worked in the Psych-Oncology Team at UCLH and in Life Force, a bereavement service in Camden & Islington. Before that, he worked with adolescents with complex needs at Oxleas House. Currently, he works in the human rights field and as a guest lecturer at the University of Hertfordshire.

Sara Portnoy is a consultant clinical psychologist who works part-time at UCLH with children who have a chronic health condition—including children with cancer—and their families. She works for Life Force, a community multidisciplinary paediatric palliative care team. The main influences on her practice are systemic and narrative theories. She developed the Beads of Life approach, a collective narrative practice, and has run many groups with young people who have a diagnosis of cancer, using this approach. She is a qualified mindfulness teacher.

PREFACE

I recall arriving at the brand new Teenage Cancer Unit of University College London Hospital (UCLH), feeling daunted by the size and the complexity of this giant organization. It is here that I began working in 2005, a move resulting from the greatly increased numbers of patients. I had previously worked as a newly qualified child and adolescent psychotherapist in the Middlesex Hospital, a much smaller building, but the birthplace of a teenage-specific cancer service.

At UCLH, the multidisciplinary team meetings held to discuss the teenage patients started to include the medical doctors, and treatments were discussed alongside each patient's psychological needs. I remember vividly my sense of "not knowing": lots of new acronyms and words that meant nothing to me, but everyone else seemed to know, spun around in meetings. Drugs that had long and often unpronounceable names that at times sounded almost poetic somehow took hold in my mind and would roll around my head like secret codes.

I felt utterly at sea, as though I had been dropped into some foreign land, as Christopher Hitchens (2012) described, although for me the strangeness was not linked to illness as it was for him. I was on the other side to those who were unwell, the side that allowed me to walk into clinics without that stomach-churning fear.

I did, of course, wonder if I had various conditions and found myself checking NHS websites for symptoms or casually asking questions of staff in those clinics. Then I feared I might catch some horrible disease by merely being in a hospital and visiting the wards. Ironically, I think that in all my years at the hospital, I had only a couple of days off for illness.

The hospital, any hospital, is a place that holds a whole range of feelings; a mix of fear, hopes, relief, joy, grief, and, of course, despair. Emotions are very raw—often exposed and palpable in the air, even if not expressed verbally or physically. My heart would begin to race when I heard a child or parent wail; I yearned to take that pain away. Sometimes I could help a little, and sometimes I had to sit and know that all I could do would be to sit and hold on to those feelings.

I had to learn to sit in a clinic with consultants and patients and hear the diagnosis, treatment, and prognosis for children and adolescents. I witnessed parents and children alike break down in shock or sometimes exclaim their relief at their treatable condition. For a time I felt useless, and then all the years of analytic training found their voice, and I realized that, of course, I, and psychoanalysis, had a place. I must hear and contain these "bombshells". I must learn to bear witness to the shock and terror that often descended: even if cure was possible, ordinary families' worlds were turned upside down in a matter of minutes. Sometimes there were tears, and sometimes there was anger at the number of times the young person had been told it was "growing pains".

Gradually I got to know the staff and began to understand more about how the hospital worked. I began to have a rudimentary knowledge of the terms used in connection with a condition. Those strange-sounding medications became more familiar, although the way they worked remained a mystery.

I discovered that some families found it comforting to talk with me, that they knew I could not take away the illness, but I could at least sit with them and hear their story. I found that many of the doctors welcomed my presence in a clinic, especially with those patients where cancer and a bad outcome might be a possibility. I came to understand the huge impact this disease has not only on patients, but on staff. It was often a relief for staff to know that I might accompany a family from the clinic to my own consulting room, where we could talk, or not, but that the family might have a moment or two to gather themselves after such shocking news—a sense that support was available, someone who could also feel the blow but be able to offer a shoulder to weep on, or someone at whom to vent their understandable but uncontrollable rage.

Over the 18 or so years that I have worked at this hospital, most of that time has been spent in the paediatric cancer division. My colleagues outside the hospital are sometimes amazed that I stayed so long, but in truth

I came to love the work. At times it would feel unbearable, and I would find myself weeping privately or experiencing uncalled-for rage as I left the hospital and entered the busy streets of London: didn't they know what was going on just up the street, in that hospital . . . ? Sometimes I would feel relief at being able to walk away. It was not me . . . it was not my child or a member of my family.

But it was about life and about death—something we all have to face, in whatever guise it appears. I felt that it was important for those of us who can bear this type of work to do it, to be alongside the doctors, nurses, and countless other professionals who work so tirelessly. It often felt an honour and privilege to work with families of amazing courage and fortitude, such as the family with whom I worked for a short period after the death of their son in hospital. The five of us would gather and talk, I would hear their stories and share their laughter and then their tears, until one day they thanked me and said that now they felt ready to take their boy, their brother, home with them. We had talked him back firmly into their hearts and minds. Their sense of having left him behind no longer plagued them. It was such a powerful moment, and I felt so privileged to have been a part of it.

There are times when things do not go so well, and one must bear the rage and hatred expressed by bereaved families or by families whose child may not have died, but who may have been permanently changed by their cancer, especially by brain tumours. At times like this it was so important to be a part of a team, to feel the support of that team: hence the evolution of the Psych-Oncology Team.

We could come together to understand the reasons and meanings of such huge emotion. We could support the medical staff who often had to hear such pain and anger first-hand. I came to understand that often there were no specific reasons for complaint other than the most profound: that their child had died or was no longer the child they had known.

This book came about as we all wanted to talk about the experiences we have had over the many years that we have worked with this extraordinary group of young people, parents, and staff.

In the chapters that follow we have written about our work with adolescent and young adult patients. We would like to thank all these young people and their families: it has been an inspiration and an honour to work with them. Some patients have generously given permission for us to use extracts from therapeutic sessions. These extracts may be an exact account of the session or conversation with their therapist. Others will just be a compilation of our work and are not about one particular patient but, rather, parts of the many events that have taught us a great deal. Throughout, however, all names and sometimes genders have been changed to protect patients' identities.

As the majority of our work is with the TYA patients seen by this service, that is what this book is about. It is for all those young people, their families and carers. It is for those who work in hospitals and clinics where this group of patients are treated.

It is difficult to see or hear about anyone diagnosed with cancer. We all have an idea of the harshness of the treatment and will, of course, often associate cancer with death. Teenagers and young people have rather particular needs that can complicate their care. There are very real medical issues that make treatment more complex.

Adolescence and young adulthood is a period in our lives when our bodies and minds are changing at a phenomenal rate. This can mean, of course, that moods fluctuate and make communication and consistent care more challenging. Adolescents may miss appointments, or seem surly and unapproachable. They can make us feel small, stupid, boring, old—as if we have no idea about what it is to be young. Many of these feelings that we experience are ones our patients may themselves be feeling but cannot express because the words are just not available to them, or they fear losing control. This might, in their minds, result in a collapse or breakdown that would be humiliating and from which there would be no return. To be in the presence of such despair and panic can be very stressful, especially if we find ourselves, out of the blue, experiencing similar emotions. It may be that in that moment we may be receiving a nonverbal communication of a patient's feelings. Knowing this can be helpful and grounding, for it can give us an insight into that patient's fears. I hope that this book, with its shared experiences, thoughts, and ideas, will also be a useful resource.

We very much hope that the chapters that follow will be of use to you in your cancer journey or in your work, because what you read either gives a different perspective or confirms what you have felt yourself. We hope that it pays tribute, too, to this small band of young people who are whipped away from their complex task of growing up and thrown into the swirling and confusing world of medicine. I have been changed by my experiences—I hope, for the better—and I do feel indebted to all the families I have met during my years at the hospital.

Introduction

Jane Elfer

This book is about the work of the Psych-Oncology Team in a large London hospital. The team is part of a larger paediatric teenage and young adult (TYA) psychological medicine service. We support children and young people and their parents when they come to the hospital for treatment for short- or long-term work.

The Psych-Oncology Team is made up of child psychotherapists, child and adolescent psychiatrists, and clinical psychologists. While much of what we do is similar, there are also unique and valuable differences, giving the team a broad spectrum of approaches for the patients.

Mike Groszmann introduces the service in greater detail in the first chapter. He gives an account of how our service emerged and sets it in the context of the growing understanding that TYA cancer requires a particular approach. He writes of how the complexity of this age group brings with it many challenges for the medical and psychological care of these patients. There are many references here that pay tribute to the enormous amount of work that is going on in this area. He describes the many different sorts of referrals we receive and shows how we manage them, with some lively vignettes.

Groszmann then writes, in chapter 2, about how our patients manage their medical treatments in a variety of ways, some of which are very challenging. The Psych-Oncology Team is especially fortunate, as we do have access to a variety of disciplines, and we have been able, as far as

DOI: 10.4324/9781003325475-1

possible, to find the right type of support for most of the young people in our care.

Then, in chapter 3, I give a more detailed description of adolescence and young adulthood as a time of enormous change that everyone goes through, sooner or later. This chapter about adolescents and young adults with cancer reminds us all to keep in mind how young people in this age group who do not have cancer might behave. This challenging period of our lives is filled with extraordinary energy and creativity but can also plunge us into feelings of despair and hopelessness. When a young person is diagnosed with cancer, this can impact their ability to do all that they might have done in healthy times, but it may not remove the urge or compulsion to do those things. This can lead to risk on a grander scale: unprotected sex while receiving chemotherapy, missing vital medications or scan appointments. A diagnosis of cancer at this time removes the young person from the support of their peers and can expose them to feelings of isolation. Their bodies are affected by the treatment in ways that we cannot prevent, and even if the changes are temporary, self-esteem can plummet. So they may take risks alone and in an angry, death-defying, or hopeless mood. It can make them hard to reach. With this in mind, we need to be flexible and to work creatively; we need to accept that the young person will choose who they talk to: it may not be us, but we can always offer support to the member of staff who does have that role.

Chapter 4 continues this line of thought as Anna Galloway, clinical psychologist, writes of the importance of keeping TYA patients connected—connected with their medical teams, but also with themselves and their emerging identities. Galloway writes about illness as "relational" and introduces her chapter thinking about our experiences with illness in this first-world country. Some young people will have heard the word "cancer" at a young age. They may have experienced a relative being unwell. Galloway notes that every young adult she has met knows about cancer and will have associated it with death. Even if the prognosis is good, that sudden and shocking connection to their mortality disrupts their "entire system" and is often what leads them to ask for a referral to the Psych-Oncology Team. Galloway, as a predominately systemic therapist, finds that it can help a young adult to begin their talking if someone else, such as a parent, partner, or nurse, is also involved. She advises a slow and gentle start to build rapport, especially as this type of talking may be a new experience.

I think that I am most struck by Galloway's adaptability. She can remain focused on what the young adult wishes to achieve but does not have a preconceived idea of how to get there. Her account of two patients shows them finding a way to live alongside their cancer and be helpful. They do not lose sight of the life that they had built for themselves, while at the same time they find ways to adapt to their changed selves. Talking about talking is especially helpful. What does the patient hope to achieve? How can this be done? It is a delicate balance, but in both cases it proved to be so important for both the patient but also the family, who must live on after the death of the young person. This type of end-of-life work is revisited in our last chapter.

Daniel Glazer, also a clinical psychologist, continues, in chapter 5, the theme of shock and trauma caused when a diagnosis of cancer is given. He uses particular approaches in neuroscience to understand the impact of trauma in relation to a diagnosis of cancer, including eye movement desensitisation and reprocessing therapy (EMDR). Glazer explains the definition of post-traumatic shock with the word "noema"—the Greek work for "a thought, judgement or perception"—as used by the nineteenth-century philosopher Edmund Husserl. Glazer invites us to think about the explosion of this noema when a diagnosis of cancer comes to a young person. He writes of the "shattering of the assumptive world", helpfully depicting how so much of that world is destroyed in one moment.

As someone trained to deliver EMDR, Glazer sees many patients who remain traumatized after their diagnosis. It is a reminder that all patients will experience their treatment differently, and he goes on to describe his work with three very different patients, including Mohamed, who shows Glazer how in the light of this devastation the end of treatment can feel like taking a penalty kick: the most important thing in the world, and so simple in one sense and in another the decider on how life will be lived in the future. Finally, he reminds us of the Japanese art of Kintsugi: the art of repairing pottery without losing the character gained from the breakage. This leads him to think about post-traumatic growth and how for some the trauma and upset of cancer can lead to a re-evaluation, which in turn can, for some, mean not only regrowth but new growth, too.

Chapter 6 continues the theme of the impact of cancer treatment, the "late effects" of life-saving but sometimes life-changing treatment. Petra Mohr, child psychotherapist, writes of the traces left behind after such an illness in infancy or early childhood. These traces leave an emotional legacy that can be reawakened in adolescence, just when a young person is attempting independence. Mohr writes of how the young people she sees can feel as if they were picked out for cancer because of what they had or had not done in an earlier life. Superstition seems to play a part—how could this happen to me? Everyone else just continues on with their lives, uninterrupted by such trauma. It can cause such a dilemma for parent and young person—who did what to whom, and why? Is it someone's fault? This can be such a haunting question, especially when sometimes the cancer takes on a persona that seems alive and vengeful. These fantasies lead also to feelings of guilt, such as her example of Chloe, who felt that the strain of her illness had such an impact on her parents that it led to their divorce. The popular image of fighting cancer with armies of chemotherapy and physical determination contributes to the feeling that cancer is some sort of malevolent being intent on causing pain and destruction, very much in the way that a country at war affects everyone.

Mohr points out that having cancer as an infant or young child has a profound impact that is felt again as the person moves in to adolescent and young adulthood. The physical and emotional experiences that are held in the body need some thoughtful processing. As Mohr reminds us, most frightening experiences in childhood can be usually be contained by a parent, but cancer in early childhood—and, indeed, in later childhood—profoundly affects not only the child, but the parents and their parenting of that child. Mohr describes how the impact of such experiences can reappear around the time of important life changes, such as puberty or leaving home to go to university. Follow-up visits can also trigger old terrors, as it does for Verity, who moves from self-harm in the form of cutting to having tattoos, despite her deep fear of needles.

The impact of childhood cancer can be far-reaching and can mean that young people have to work out a narrative to tell friends that fills in the missing months or years of their childhood without telling them about their cancer. They may also feel that they themselves have little memory of that childhood drama. They must piece that life together using fragments of memory or what they have been told by parents. Psychological support for this group is so helpful and, in the team's experience, responded to well.

Chapter 7, by Claudia Henry, a child psychotherapist, is about hope. Henry reminds us of the Greek myth of Pandora's Box but also tells of a detail that can be overlooked alongside the more dramatic escape of the horrors. Hope, a small but beautiful dragonfly, emerges when the box appears empty. She also reminds us that some of our work takes place in the midst of trauma, when often hope seems to have flown away. Conversely when the prognosis is poor, any feelings of hope can be misinterpreted. Henry recalls an Italian saying that "Hope is the last thing to die", and this seems to link with an extraordinary capacity in some young people and their families to remain "in the moment", looking only at having a "good" day, for example.

Henry explores the complexity of working with young people who feel "hopeless" but who can, with family support or a member of the Psych-Oncology Team, find often unknown resources deep inside. She helpfully uses Donald Meltzer's 1994 paper on temperature and distance, which seems so apt in a medical setting. Henry writes about sitting alongside, listening and taking in meaning and feeling, which is similar to what Galloway also describes. The therapist may have an urgent feeling or wish to do something, to make it better, or, as Henry so honesty writes, "I have a familiar feeling of wanting to be elsewhere . . .". The strength of emotions faced by staff is powerful, and if these feelings are not recognized as projections from the patient or family, it can result in a flight to action or a reason not to visit. Henry is able to think and to enable a mother to draw herself together, to be strong, but only, I believe, because the mother knows that Henry understands this need within her. In the light of these powerful feelings, Henry concludes with some thoughts about how the Psych-Oncology Team might support staff who are with families daily and on long shifts.

Fittingly, in chapter 8, James McParland, Cristian Pena, and Sara Portnoy generously allow us to sit in on a conversation they had about death: "a sensitive topic to cover, we conclude, and many people prefer to avoid the topic altogether". The feeling that the death of someone young goes against nature describes, I think, the struggle that is perhaps more present in the death of a young person. There is the sense of all the potential in adolescence and young adulthood, perhaps, I wonder, bound up with an idea of fertility, which is so often the marker for moving into that period of our lives. The authors struggle to find a way to work with families who face the death of a young person in a way that is authentic for each patient, even if it is informed by important theories—work that is vital if that young patient is to feel that they can discuss their complex feelings at this time.

The importance of the patient's close relationships seems to be echoed by this trio's own trust in speaking together openly. Portnoy quotes Bergum and Dossetor (2005), who wrote of the importance of "mutual respect", among other things, and as these clinicians speak I have a sense of this, and that this enables them to work closely with families in these difficult times with respect and "heart". They write powerfully of the young person perhaps losing sight of who they are as they enter such frightening and unfamiliar territory—that "liminal" place, as McParland describes. Using the Beads of Life (Portnoy, Girling, & Fredman, 2016) can help patients describe who they were before illness and in this way regain something of their history.

Pena speaks of "chronic sorrow": the young person can lose sight of who they are and can begin to feel unreal. He helpfully reminds us that this is not pathological, but a very reasonable response. The authors also write about hope—of "holding on to hope" and "reasonable hope" and how being able to be available and "truly present" enables these "hopes" to be understood, not only as a wish, but as a state of mind. Families might be able to "do" certain things together as a way of managing the time available to them.

Pena writes that "you cannot tame death", and the three authors acknowledge that there is no "getting over" the loss of a child. Families must find a way to live alongside their grief, that grief does not get smaller but life expands around it. The chapter ends with some thoughts about self-care, of the importance of having a good team around you and feeling able to use this support. This is a fitting end to the book, as it highlights the value of a good and close team, one that can function because they are open to difference and value their colleagues' opinions.

Our hope, therefore, is that our experiences and thoughts will be of use to all who read this book. We have learnt so much from the families we have worked with and have a debt of gratitude to them and to all our colleagues alongside whom we worked.

CHAPTER ONE

Overview:
cancer in teenagers and young adults
and psycho-oncology

Mike Groszmann

Adolescents and young adults have been described as a "lost tribe" of cancer patients (McCabe, 2018). Until relatively recently, treatment was crudely divided between paediatric and adult services, leaving young people in a "no man's land" of shortcomings in communication, in clinical ethos, in collaboration, and in transitions (Hollis & Morgan, 2001). Adolescents 16 years old and older were treated on adult wards, surrounded by older and often elderly patients they felt different from, observing frailty, severe sickness, and exposure to death (Bleyer, 2002; Bleyer, Morgan, & Barr, 2006; McCabe, 2018). For many, this made an already terrifying experience enter the realms of horror. They experienced isolation from peers, little opportunity for age-appropriate activities, and no opportunity for ongoing education. Younger adolescents, under 16 years, were treated on paediatric wards surrounded by babies and much younger children, with "kiddie" décor and activities that were experienced as inappropriate and unappealing. They were nursed and treated by teams unfamiliar with the distinct types of cancer affecting this age group and often lacking the particular skills and approaches that make clinical care more accessible, acceptable, and therefore more effective for adolescents and young adults (Albritton, Caligiuri, Anderson, & Nichols, 2006; NICE, 2005). Historically, children and young people would spend a great deal of time in hospital during cancer treatment—this could mean many months on the ward, with little time at home, in school, or with peers. Accordingly, while treatment outcomes and cancer survival rates improved dramatically for younger children (Benowitz, 2000) and older persons (National Cancer Institute, 2001, 2022), improvements were far more modest for teenagers and young adults (Bleyer & Barr, 2007).

The experience of being diagnosed and treated for cancer as a young person in England has been transformed in many ways, however. A distinct concept of teenage and young adult (TYA—preferred in the United Kingdom) or adolescent and young adult (AYA—preferred in the United States, Europe, and Australia) cancer gained prominence in the 2000s, when professional concern was supported by various national initiatives and service changes (McCabe, 2018; Stark & Ferrari, 2018). Only relatively recently have the improvements in outcomes begun to approach those seen in younger and older cancer patient populations (Barr, Ferrari, Ries, & Whelan, 2016; Keegan, Ries, Barr, & Geiger, 2016; O'Hara, Moran, Whelan, & Hough, 2015; Stark, Bielack, & Brugieres, 2016), though there remain significant disparities (McCabe, 2018; Stark & Ferrari, 2018). The reasons for this are complex, varied, and still not fully understood. These include longer intervals between signs or symptoms and diagnosis, resulting in later diagnosis and more progressive disease at the point of starting treatment (Cancer Research UK, 2021; Fern, Birch, Whelan, Cooke, & Sutton, 2013; Lyratzopoulos, Neal, Barbiere, Rubin, & Abel, 2012). There is greater physiological sensitivity in young people to side-effects, making treatments even more difficult to tolerate (Rugbjerg & Olsen, 2016; Rugbjerg, Mellemkjaer, & Boice, 2014). Some of the particular types of cancers affecting this age group have worse prognoses—especially central nervous system (brain and spinal cord) tumours, sarcomas (soft tissue and bone cancers), and particular haematological malignancies (Tricoli, Blair, Anders, & Bleyer, 2016). Psychosocial factors are also significant and affect treatment acceptance and concordance (Morgan, Davies, Palmer, & Plaster, 2010; Zebrack, 2011), adolescence and young-adulthood being a phase where there are commonly challenges to authority, conformity, and convention that conflicts with the relatively conservative and hierarchical medical establishment. Treatment competes with other more pressing priorities, such as peer activities, academic progress (exams, university), employment, gaining independence, and leaving the family home. Additionally, relatively less research has been undertaken into this group, with poor levels of recruitment to existing clinical trials, as well as a relative paucity of clinical trials specifically for this age group (Bleyer, Budd, & Montello, 2005; Bleyer et al., 1997; Fern & Whelan, 2018).

Changes over the last 20 years in how and where TYA are treated are beginning to improve clinical outcomes (Keegan et al., 2016; O'Hara et al.,

2015; Stark & Ferrari, 2018). TYA patients appear to have better outcomes when treatment is delivered in an age-appropriate setting, alongside other young people—perhaps because they are more likely to accept and adhere to treatment (Stark & Ferrari, 2018). Young people who are physically well enough to do so might "ambulate", attending hospital for the day to receive chemotherapy and returning home or to a local hospital-provided hotel for the night, sometimes even taking their treatment away from hospital in a "back-pack" that continues to deliver the intravenous treatments away from the hospital (McMonagle, 2018). The aim is to maximize patients' normalcy, retain as much of their pre-cancer life as possible, and for them to experience the typical rites of passage. There is greater appreciation of the impact when this not possible, so it can be responded to more helpfully. This can better enable young people to reach their developmental milestones, despite the setbacks that a cancer diagnosis can impose (Morgan et al., 2010). Hospital schools allow young people to continue their studies if they are well enough to do so, and they can liaise with a patient's school, college, or university, allowing them to feel slightly less isolated from their peers and from their progress in their occupation (Hollis & Morgan, 2001). These innovations are increasingly available in England from specialist TYA Cancer Primary Treatment Centres, as part of Specialist Commissioning of Cancer Services by NHS-England (Carr, Whiteson, Edwards, & Morgan, 2013; NICE, 2005). Despite this, there are still teenagers and young adults with cancer who do not receive treatment in this setting or by these specialist teams, depending on where they are seen and what they are being treated for (Stark & Ferrari, 2018).

Cancer statistics

According to the Cancer Research report on teenage and young adult cancer (Cancer Research UK, 2021), cancer is the leading cause of disease-related death in teenagers and young adults in the United Kingdom: around 2,200 15–24-year-olds are diagnosed with cancer each year, and around 310 die from it. According to a World Health Organization report (WHO, 2021), world-wide approximately 400,000 children aged 0–19 years are diagnosed with cancer each year. Mortality rates for all cancers combined have almost halved since the mid-1970s, though incidence rates have increased over the same period. In Europe and the United States, the overall five-year survival rates of TYA cancer patients have exceeded 80%, with improvements in some haematological malignancies and other diverse cancers in the last 20 years due to TYA cancer innovations. There have, however, been no such improvements in survival rates for other cancers, such as high-grade glioma brain-tumours and certain bone or soft-tissue sarcomas. About a quarter of TYA cancer patients present to hospitals requiring emergency medical admission, which suggests that they present late, with more progressive disease (Cancer Research UK, 2021; McCabe, 2018).

Psychological support in cancer treatment

Psychological and psychosocial support is widely recognized as being of key importance in meeting the holistic needs of TYA who have or have had cancer (Holland & Thompson, 2018; Kazak & Noll, 2015; Mooney, Jacobson, Chesman, & Mann, 2016; NICE, 2005). Various guidelines (such as London Cancer, 2014; Macmillan Cancer Support, 2013; Mooney et al., 2016; NICE, 2005, 2014; Wiener, Kazak, Noll, Patenaude, & Kupst, 2015) recommend that psychological support is important and should be a routine part of a cancer multidisciplinary team (MDT). The psychological impact of the illness and its treatment can be significant, varied, and wide-reaching (CLIC Sargent, 2017; McCarthy et al., 2016; Steele, Mullins, Mullins, & Muriel, 2015). Typically, this can include adjustment reactions, such as anxiety, depression, panic, and/or distress, procedural anxiety, or phobia of components of treatment, such as needles, swallowing tablets, scans, or the hospital itself (Datta, Cardona, Mahanta, Younus, & Lax-Pericall, 2019; McFarland & Holland, 2017), and anticipatory nausea or other symptoms that precede and complicate treatment (Kazak & Noll, 2015). Some have direct neuropsychiatric or other physical causes, with psychiatric symptoms, resulting from direct brain pathology—for example, in cases of brain tumours or central nervous system inflammation as a side-effect of chemotherapy (Datta et al., 2019). Over the arduous and frightening course of treatment, patients can become depressed or significantly "demoralized" (Kissane, 2017); they may suffer with traumatic stress or post-traumatic stress disorder (Bruce, Gumley, Isham, & Fearon, 2011; Datta et al., 2019; Holland & Thompson, 2018).

The National Institutes of Health (NIH) National Cancer Institute (NCI) defines "late effect" as:

> A health problem that occurs months or years after a disease is diagnosed or after treatment has ended. Late effects may be caused by cancer or cancer treatment. They may include physical, mental, social problems and secondary cancers. [NCI, 2020]

There is increasing recognition of the cognitive and psychological late effects experienced by patients cured of their cancer (Ahmad, Reinius,

Hatcher, Ajithkumar, 2016; Barnett et al., 2016; Pitman, Suleman, Hyde, & Hodgkiss, 2018). The social consequences of cancer, its treatment, and its late effects are also increasingly recognized (CLIC Sargent, 2013, 2014, 2016; Holland & Thompson, 2018; Schulte et al., 2018). All children, teen-agers, and young adults diagnosed with cancer in England are eligible for the formerly-known CLIC Sargent (recently renamed "Young Lives vs Cancer") social support for patients and their families. In our hospi-tal every patient is offered an allocated charity (Young Lives vs Cancer) social worker (CLIC Sargent, 2013, 2014). They are also allocated a TYA cancer clinical nurse specialist (CNS) who coordinates and offers consist-ency to the young person and their family throughout treatment (NICE, 2005, 2014). Alongside the medical team, ward, or day-care nursing team and allied health professionals, they provide basic (so-called "Level 1–2") psychological support to patients encountering "normal" levels of dis-tress during treatment (Mooney et al., 2016; NICE, 2005, 2014). When this is not sufficient, or when cancer patients have significant pre-existing mental health difficulties, more specialist mental health interventions and support are needed ("Level 3–4") as part of a well-functioning, holistic multidisciplinary cancer team (Holland & Thompson, 2018; Mooney et al., 2016). There are various recommendations for what this specialist ser-vice could or should entail, in terms of professional disciplines and avail-able interventions (Macmillan Cancer Support, 2013; Mooney et al., 2016; NICE, 2005, 2014; Wiener et al., 2015).

The majority of the literature on psycho-oncology—or psychosocial oncology—relates to treatment of adults (e.g., Holland, 2018; Holland et al., 2015; Kissane, 2022), though there is a growing body of literature on paediatric, adolescent, and young-adult psycho-oncology (e.g., Datta et al., 2019; Holland & Thompson, 2018; Seitz, Besier, & Goldbeck, 2009; Wiener, Pao, Kazak, Kupst, & Patenaude, 2014). In large oncology centres there may be dedicated psycho-oncology professionals—usually psychologists and sometimes some psychiatrists, psychotherapists, and/or counselling professionals, as well as mental health/liaison nurses—but this tends to be the exception. Most services will have some level of access to psycholo-gists, either within the service or from a psychology team that extends to the cancer service. In adult cancer centres, psychological treatment is often accessed through an associated wider supportive service, usually run by a charity, such as Macmillan (Macmillan Cancer Support, 2021) or Maggie's (www.maggies.org/our-centre). Specialist services may commission spe-cialist psycho-oncology professionals, such as dedicated liaison psychia-trists and/or mental health nurses, neuropsychologists, neuropsychiatrists, and therapists. Unfortunately, many services and cancer patients still have extremely limited—if any—access to specialist psychological or psychiatric interventions. This is particularly true internationally and in developing countries (CCLG, 2021) and remains a significant area for development.

There are different models for the delivery of psychological support to patients with cancer (Fann & Sexton, 2015). Most emphasize that cancer is not a mental illness, and that therefore the majority of children and young people *will not need* the involvement of a mental health professional, irrespective of whether or not they might benefit from one (Mooney et al., 2016; NICE, 2005, 2014). Young people and their parents have sometimes complained to our team that having a cancer diagnosis is difficult enough as it is; they really do not want to consider a mental health difficulty on top of this. This sentiment probably relates in part to the all-consuming nature of cancer and its treatment, sometimes leaving little room for patients and their families to consider other aspects of health. The ongoing stigma around mental health might add to this reticence, however, and can be a barrier to receiving psychological support (CLIC Sargent, 2017; Naylor et al., 2012). The recent national James Lind Alliance Research Priority Setting Programme for TYA patients found that the *highest priority* for future research was, according to patients, their families, and clinicians, to investigate effective interventions to improve the psychological/mental health of this patient group (Aldiss et al., 2019). Rarely, services have a psychologist routinely present alongside the oncologist and oncology nurse when a cancer diagnosis is shared with a family. This carries a significant cost and resource implication, however, which makes the model untenable currently within NHS services, despite arguments for its benefits. At our hospital, there is an ethos that only those patients with significant emotional, psychological, or behavioural difficulties are referred to the Psych-Oncology Team for specialist mental health assessments and interventions, though patients who request input are usually offered at least assessment. Non-specialist, so-called "Level 1 & 2", support (Macmillan Cancer Support, 2013; Mooney et al., 2016; NICE, 2005) can be provided by other members of the team—usually medical/nursing staff from oncology or symptom control and palliative care teams, oncology CNSs, play specialists or activity coordinators, physiotherapists, occupational therapists, and Young Lives vs Cancer social workers. We have seen, however, that when there are staff shortages, or when levels of anxiety in staff are high, more referrals tend to be directed to the Psych-Oncology Team, even when the need for specialist intervention is not necessarily apparent.

The evolution of the Psych-Oncology Team

Prior to about 2010, there was no separate team or service supporting oncology patients. They were referred to the psychological medicine/psychology team within the hospital paediatric department and seen by whichever discipline was available or seemed most suitable. The first step towards a more dedicated team came from a psychiatrist and psychotherapist committing to consistently attending the oncology MDT meeting, where most referrals were made during case discussion, and referrals tended to be seen and managed by these individuals. A psychologist with specialist neuropsychology experience was involved in neurocognitive assessments for children and young people with brain tumours or cranio-spinal radiation treatment, and often joined the psychosocial MDT meetings. With publication of the NICE guidelines (NICE, 2005, 2014) and Macmillan standards (Macmillan Cancer Support, 2013), and when cancer services became specially commissioned by NHS England (NICE, 2014), involvement of psychological support by mental health professionals was needed for Best Practice tariffs and became a requirement in the regular peer reviews and clinical reference groups (Stark & Ferrari, 2018). At our hospital, from about 2011 onwards, a child and adolescent psychiatrist, a child and adolescent psychotherapist, and a clinical psychologist met after the weekly psychosocial MDT meetings to discuss cases and to allocate clinical work. As the oncology service tripled in size, more referrals were made, and additional psychologists and psychotherapists were allocated to work with cancer patients and their families. In 2014, the three disciplines came together to develop a standard operational policy and referral and treatment pathways, and they implemented a regular meeting to discuss referrals, allocate cases, develop the team, and learn together. And so the Children, Teenage and Young Adult Psych-Oncology Team came into being!

Team name

The team is referred to in a number of different ways by patients and referrers. These include "counselling"/"counsellors", the "psychology team" or "psych team", or "mental health", or reference is made to the particular individual a patient sees (psychologist, psychotherapist, psychiatrist). For some time we referred to ourselves as the "psycho-oncology team" but found that "psycho" had rather negative and off-putting connotations. We discussed our name with patients and the wider MDT, all of whom preferred "psych-oncology", and so, in about 2016, Psych-Oncology Team was chosen as the preferred title.

The multidisciplinary psycho-oncology approach

As a team, we recognize and appreciate the broad range of experience as well as clinical approaches that each team member, and each discipline, brings to the table. Psycho-oncology is a relatively new field of work, with peculiarities and particularities, some of which cross over to other areas of "paediatric liaison"/health psychology (psychological work in physical illness)/child and adolescent psychotherapy in applied-settings, and others that are relatively unique.

The team

Our team consists of child and adolescent psychotherapists trained in the psychoanalytic/psychodynamic model accredited by the Association of Child Psychotherapists (ACP); clinical psychologists with specialist experience of work with children, adolescents, and families and trained to use a combination of systemic family therapy, narrative therapy, health psychology, motivational interviewing, and cognitive behavioural therapy (CBT) models; and psychiatrists trained in the bio-psychosocial and medical models. Each discipline has a slightly different approach, emphasis, and preferred explanatory model, but there are many commonalities and "generic skills" that are shared and overlap.

Psychotherapists tend to be less structured and task- or symptom-focused and, rather, making use of sensitive and attuned enquiry, careful observation, and paying attention to unconscious communications as well as what is explicitly described. Initial meetings may follow a formal psychodynamic State of Mind assessment (Mees, 2017) or be informed by this assessment approach. Psychotherapists attend to the quality of the relationship formed, using the *transference* (aspects of a patient's key previous relationships that impact how they relate to and experience others) and *countertransference* (the feelings that are evoked in the therapist when relating to their patient) as additional communications that can aid a deeper level of understanding of what a patient might share. Younger children may use toys, play, or drawing as an alternative to verbal communication, whereas adolescents and adults would usually not use these "props". Sessions tend to be patient-led, and therapists aim to offer as much consistency as possible in a hospital setting, to enable the therapeutic space to become the place where a patient's internal psychological world can be understood.

Psychologists tend to be more explicit and structured and may take a more active, guiding role in assessments and treatment. They will identify and seek to understand the perspectives of their patient/client and those of key people in their lives, such as parents/family, clinicians, teachers, friends, and so on. There is a focus on goals, strengths, capabilities, and hopes as well as problems or difficulties. There is an attempt to "be with" the patient/client/family member and their experience. Metaphor is often used to find a shared language and understanding of what is experienced. Solutions may be more explicitly sought and worked on—varying from suggested practical exercises or things to try to agreed "homework", such as "behavioural experiments" and "thought diaries" if using a CBT model. Work may include direct work with the individual or the parents/family, or in a group. Creative approaches may be employed, such as using beads to tell their story and share their experience (see chapter 8).

Psychiatrists undertake an assessment that focuses on particular symptoms or difficulties, seeking to identify whether there are features of a psychiatric condition, and to understand these in the bio-psychosocial context of their patients. They seek to develop a formulation that can guide potential interventions directed at the individual, their family, or their social circle. They routinely assess and manage risks. Whereas the commonest interventions used are psychological and/or social, psychiatrists can prescribe medications where appropriate; they have expertise in how physical illness and treatments can impact the mind; and they are able to make use of the various legal frameworks that may be required to ensure that patients receive treatments and that their safety is maintained.

All three disciplines require excellent listening and communication skills, adopting a non-judgemental position of curiosity and compassion, and having the ability to focus on the key relationships and develop these. By not directly delivering cancer treatments, psycho-oncology clinicians are better-placed to take up a position alongside patients or their families that can enable their perspective to be heard, understood, and communicated. All three disciplines attend to risks and take responsibility for safety and safeguarding, working together to protect patients, their families, and staff. In this sense, these professionals have more in common than not. Moreover, individual clinicians have diverse experiences, interests, and skills, which often cross disciplinary boundaries. For example, our psychiatrist has training and experience in psychodynamic and systemic psychotherapies. Our psychologists value psychodynamic formulations and interpretations. Our psychotherapists find the group work, family work, and the more structured approach of a systemic model invaluable for patients who may struggle to make use of psychodynamic therapy. All disciplines have found value in mindfulness practices to complement other interventions, as well as being a helpful intervention in itself.

Cancer and its treatment can be all-consuming for patients and their families, and it affects different people in different ways. A high degree of flexibility is needed to adapt assessments, offer support, and deliver interventions to patients and their families' circumstances, making allowances for sickness, disabilities, treatments, investigations, and the wholly unpredictable and uncertain nature of the course of disease and treatments (Datta et al., 2019; Holland & Thompson, 2018).

Team processes

From referral to first contact

Our team meets weekly to discuss and process new referrals. Each referral is presented to the team, to allow reflections and hypotheses to be made. Where sufficient information is available, we decide as a team who would be most suitable to contact the referred patient/client. Ideally, whenever possible, this decision is based on the particular challenges a patient faces and which approach/skill-set seems best suited to address this. Our clinical psychologists make initial contact using a "relationship to help" semi-structured interview, based on a paper by Reder and Fredman (1996). This is an initial conversation with a referred patient to explore what they hope to achieve by receiving support. The patient can talk about what has been helpful in the past and what has not been helpful. The clinician and patient can then think together about the best way to proceed with the offer of "help". Other members of the team, while not necessarily using this model formally, will make initial contact with similar enquiries. Whose idea was it to see our team? Who is most worried and why? We establish whether the referred patient *actually wants to receive help* from the team, or whether this is what their parent or clinical team thinks is needed. We explore what help might look like, what help has been offered before, and how this help was experienced. If a positive experience, what was it they appreciated? If negative, what made it so? It is not uncommon that a parent, sibling, or another professional believes that a young person "needs" psychological support—usually for very good and well-intentioned reasons—but this may not correspond with what the young person wants themselves. Working psychologically is practically impossible when there is no buy-in from the person you are trying to work with. There are very few situations where anything useful can be done against a patient's will, and it can be counterproductive to push them. Helping a young person get to the point of accepting psychological support can be an important intervention in itself, those around them taking the time and making the effort to help to shift them to the point of help-seeking (see Vignettes 1, 4, & 5). In these instances, work with a young person can shift to understanding why others are so concerned, and what can be done to make them less so. Alternatively, offering support to the concerned other—sometimes to staff, or to the patient's parent or significant other—is the best way forward, working "through" the professional or their relative/partner as a means of developing understanding and delivering help "by proxy".

The following three clinical vignettes illustrate ways to work with a young person when individual therapy is not accepted or effective.

Vignette 1. Enabling individual therapy through parent therapy: Kunle

Kunle was a 14-year-old male who had recently completed treatment for Hodgkin's lymphoma. He became withdrawn; he argued with family and avoided friends and school, preferring to stay at home in his room on his own. His parents requested psychological support, but Kunle would not agree to meet with anyone. His parents were offered appointments, but they felt they were too busy, having returned to work, and did not consider this worth while unless Kunle was there himself. They preferred to wait until they could persuade him to change his mind. He was referred again six weeks later, after a clinic review, but again Kunle refused, and the referral did not proceed. A third referral was made six months later, when little had changed, and his parents felt increasingly desperate. After gently pointing out that their reluctance to attend might be enabling or even reinforcing Kunle's refusal, his parents attended a session with a psychologist. A picture emerged of the family roles having changed dramatically over the course of Kunle's treatment. Kunle had a particularly frightening, intense treatment course, which the whole family tried to avoid remembering, as it always brought them to tears. Kunle's parents accepted psychological support for themselves, to help them process his treatment and the upsetting memories associated with it, and began monthly appointments. At their third appointment Kunle agreed to join, with the assurance that this was to help his parents and "not all about me". He appreciated that the psychologist was true to her word and maintained the focus on his parents. He found the session helpful and agreed to attend again. After a few sessions he asked to be seen individually and was able to receive his own support. This enabled him to understand his avoidance and irritability as a response to his fears—something that his family also employed to evade distress. Kunle and his parents began to face and engage with each other's distress without the previous avoidance, making the family closer and their home more harmonious and allowing him to return to school and to socialize again.

Vignette 2. Working through a parent: Jen

Jen, a 15-year-old female with Hodgkin's lymphoma, felt fearful, withdrawn, miserable, low in mood, and distressed following the combination of severe chemotherapy-related side-effects and high doses of steroids. She gained a lot of weight because of the steroids and lost her hair as a result of chemotherapy, so she felt extremely self-conscious. She hid under her covers and avoided all but essential contact. She adamantly refused to speak to anyone new, including anyone from the Psych-Oncology Team. A psychotherapist met with her mother, Patricia, who also felt desperate and wanted the team to use stealth, deceit, the Mental Health Act—frankly anything—to help Jen, none of which were professional or appropriate. Having gently explained this, it was possible to engage with Patricia's desperation and helplessness. They considered whether this might be a communication of how Jen was feeling and suggested that Patricia could share this experience with her daughter and acknowledge how awful this felt. Patricia was taken aback, having felt up to then that she needed to encourage "positivity" and recovery and reinforce a message that "everything will be ok". It became clear that, for both Patricia and Jen, frightening, helpless thoughts and feelings had to be hidden and left unspoken. Patricia believed that she needed to "be strong" and never cry in front of Jen. These beliefs were gently challenged. Patricia was helped to broach these with Jen, and they were gradually able to share their respective fears and feelings and to cry together; Patricia comforted Jen. Jen emerged from her covers and began to re-engage with her world. She maintained that she would not meet with anyone from the Psych-Oncology Team, but in fact she didn't need to, finding the understanding from her mum and their shared experience sufficient to manage her situation.

Vignette 3. Working through staff: Kiran

Kiran, a 17-year-old male with a soft-tissue tumour, struggled with more than the usual pain with this cancer and treatment. He became upset with his nurses and physiotherapists when they persistently encouraged him to shower and remain physically active between treatments. He had increasingly frequent furious outbursts, followed by upset, withdrawal, and oppositional responses. He experienced incontinence in his bed and demanded, in a hostile manner, to be cleaned up, making staff assume it was done deliberately and was experienced as an attack or retaliation. He was referred to the Psych-Oncology Team, accepted being seen, but insisted there was "nothing wrong" with him and repeatedly remonstrated about staff believing he was "mental". He used sessions to complain about individual nurses and how they were mistreating him. This persecuted position was also taken up by his parents.

It seemed clear that there was a displacement of their fears, distress, and anger around the cancer and its treatment, which was being located in staff and the relationship with them. Rather than Kiran and his parents being angry and upset about the cancer and trusting that the clinical team sought to relieve his experience and treat this alongside them, they felt that staff were angry with him/them and in opposition. Adverse symptoms were experienced as poor care or even as punishment by staff. Attempts to explore this way of understanding their experience were rejected, however. Kiran accepted seeing a psychologist ("you're the only one on my side"), but the perspectives did not shift, and at best therapy was not helping, or possibly making things worse by reinforcing his animosity. Instead of persevering with therapy, time was spent with staff instead, making sense of what was being played out and considering how staff could respond in a sensitive, informed way, holding clear but not punitive boundaries without exacerbating problems. This enabled Kiran to receive his treatment and staff to cope with looking after him.

Once it is clear a patient is on board, the team aim to explore what they are struggling with, and how it manifests. We try to get a sense, when possible, of their concerns, fears, ideas, or the basis of their difficulty. Usually this arises in the context of their illness; or difficulties in key relationships—with family, partners, peers, hospital staff, and sometimes themselves. We try to develop a *formulation*—a framework of the various factors contributing to the situation that guides understanding and intervention—and some hypotheses about the difficulties and how these might be addressed. We see whether there is a preference for whom they will see: male or female, younger or older, a particular discipline or a particular approach? While there is not always an option to meet their preferences, it is helpful to at least consider what is preferred and how characteristics of the professional will affect engagement. We establish what days, times, and frequency a patient and/or their family can manage. If still on treatment, we explore what their cancer treatment entails. Some people are referred who live very far from the hospital. Others have such intensive treatment and feel so unwell from it that regular psychological work is simply not practical. All this will inform if, with whom, how, and when we might initiate treatment, in order to be most effective.

Prior to the COVID-19 pandemic, all clinical work was done face to face, sometimes interspersed with telephone calls. Since the pandemic, video and phone appointments have been routinely offered as alternatives, and this has enabled remote working. This has improved convenience and accessibility for those able to make use of these, though it has also introduced new challenges and created greater demands for the team.

Reflections from first contact

After the initial contact, we bring back our impressions and experiences to the team, where these are discussed and other team-members' ideas are shared. These discussions are the real "gold" of our multidisciplinary working. Insights and understanding from different models and perspectives are considered, which can help enormously in making progress with our patients. Bringing a range of models, challenging preconceived ideas, and sharing different approaches to the situation opens up how difficulties can be understood and ways to intervene. The team decides who is able and best placed to proceed with supporting the young person, and how this might be approached.

The first contact is highly significant, and it is impossible to overemphasize how carefully this should be done—this may be the first time this young person or family member opens up about something deeply personal and intimate. If done clumsily, if too much is shared too soon, or if a patient feels offended, judged, or misunderstood, one risks losing the possibility of working with this young person or family member at the time, and sometimes also in the future. They may regret having opened up at all and may refuse any support in the future.

Ideally, the person making the first contact would be able to continue to offer support and treatment, if this goes well. In practice, with limited staffing and time constraints, this is not always possible. Whoever has capacity to make the initial contact will either call or meet the referred patient or family member, introduce the team, and tentatively explore the present, the past, expectations for the future, and the types of support that might help. Not uncommonly, however, it becomes clearer from the first contact who might be suited to working with the patient/family, and, when possible, this is organized. First contact can be made by phone, videoclinic, or in person, and it is important that some preparation and care is invested in making the contact positive, to avoid scuppering the meeting from the outset.

Progressing with treatment

Occasionally it only becomes clear after a few sessions what a patient needs—perhaps when a particular approach does not suit, or a patient and a therapist do not quite gel. In this instance, a clinician will bring a patient for discussion with the team, and some understanding of what is going on is established. Sometimes it is possible to "stick with" and work through the difficulties within the therapy, and resolution comes from reconciling these; indeed, this can be a critical "watershed" in treatment. In other cases, it is clear that the approach or relationship does not match or is not experienced as therapeutic, and an alternative approach and/ or therapist may need to be found. In some cases, psychological therapy is not possible at that time, and we offer patients our details, so they can self-refer or request referral in the future, should they feel that this may be more helpful at a later date.

Vignette 4. The need to change clinicians, approach, and teams in treatment: Clem

Clem was a young adult referred by the Late Effects Clinic for severe emotional distress and concerns about safety. He had received cancer treatment as a teenager on an adult cancer ward. The experience of the treatment was extremely traumatic and haunting, though he did not talk much about this at the time, desperate to just "get on with it" and complete treatment. Despite his cancer being treated successfully, and despite being a highly intelligent A* student, Clem struggled academically. He got into university but dropped out. He repeatedly found himself in situations that were unmanageable or destructive. He took up an opportunity to study abroad but made extremely risky choices, which placed him in danger. When he injured himself seriously, he returned home to recover, but he became depressed. He attended an oncology Late Effects Clinic appointment around this time and agreed to a referral to the Psych-Oncology Team.

Clem initially met with a psychotherapist on three occasions. He struggled to manage exploring aspects of himself and his past, becoming emotionally overwhelmed and "dissociating" in the room (appearing completely detached and "in another world"). He agreed to a psychiatrist joining the appointment, who diagnosed post-traumatic stress disorder and prescribed medication to help alleviate the severity of distress, which was preventing making progress, with psychological support. Over subsequent appointments, traumatic memories were shared, though Clem felt increasingly unsafe afterwards. We discussed the case within the Psych-Oncology Team meeting and agreed that a psychodynamic approach was not possible at that time. We offered a more directed trauma-focused therapy with a psychologist, alongside ongoing psychiatric treatment.

Clem was not able to engage with the psychologist, however, and became riskier and more distressed. A referral was made to the local community mental health crisis team, to manage risks more comprehensively, with more frequent appointments nearer to home and out-of-hours home treatment when needed. It became clear that Clem needed a specialist traumatic-stress service, who could work closely with his community mental health team, crisis team, and care-coordinator. He continued to see a psychiatrist within the Psych-Oncology Team until his care was taken over by the local team.

The clinical task began with assessing and offering psychological intervention, then diagnosing and treating Clem's mental disorder. When it was not
possible for him to use what the Psych-Oncology Team could offer without
excessive risk, a service offering more intensive, specialist treatment locally
was sought. The work became making a robust referral that incorporated
our understanding of the role cancer played and what was revealed during
treatment. We supported Clem to accept and access this care and "held"
him while waiting for this to start. This highlights the value of having a range
of disciplines within a Psych-Oncology Team, while recognizing the remit and
limits of what can be offered within this sort of service.

During team meetings, clinicians will bring back a case they are working
with for discussion if progress gets stuck, if anxieties in either clinician or
patient heighten, if risks escalate, or new problems emerge. The multidisciplinary nature of the team, and the resources of experience and shared
clinical skills, can often bring insights and understanding that allow
resolution and progress. Team members may suggest particular questions, lines of enquiry, ways of thinking and understanding, or creative
approaches to work with a challenge. This can often shine fresh light on
previously unrecognized elements, which helps patient and therapist in
navigating the uncertainties faced.

Vignette 5. The process of finding the right therapist and approach: Pria

Pria, a young adult with a pre-existing personality disorder, was diagnosed
with a potentially curable bone cancer. She had spoken to nurses about
death, which they understood as suicidal thoughts, and they requested urgent
psychiatric assessment. During this assessment Pria shared her preoccupation with thoughts about dying; however, these were not suicidal wishes but,
rather, distress about her potential death. She saw this as an abandoning of
her family and partner, which would cause them pain, and this she found
tormenting. Pria said her mother was also struggling, and things were tense
between them. She agreed to meet a psychologist from the team to consider psychological therapies for her and perhaps her mum. We discussed the
assessment at the Psych-Oncology meeting and hypothesized that anxieties
around loss, rejection, and abandonment might be prominent in the work.
We thought Pria might be sensitive to feeling rejected by the professionals
she meets. Trust, consistency, and regularity of appointments can help contain
these anxieties, so we thought carefully about whom she would see and
when and where she would be seen, in order to best enable these.

At the second meeting with the same male psychiatrist and a male psychologist, she was more guarded and reticent. She was seen briefly with her

mother, and then individually. She minimized her distress and said things were "fine". We offered regular appointments with the psychologist, who could more reliably offer consistency. The psychiatrist offered to remain involved and support her mother. Pria seemed troubled by this suggestion and replied, "You know my mum is married!" It was not possible to think about this further with Pria in that meeting, beyond concrete assurances and clarification. Unsurprisingly, she did not agree to see either psychologist or psychiatrist again, politely explaining that she felt too unwell from chemotherapy and later that she didn't need this any more.

The team hypothesized that the intimacy of making a psychological connection might get confused with a more sordid intimacy, and that Pria may find it easier to see a female. Perhaps psychological support needed to focus on practical, "surface-level" areas, to get started? We considered that Pria may envy her relatively young, attractive, healthy mother while she herself struggled with feeling ill and unattractive while receiving treatment. We recognized the feelings of rejection that may have been stirred up by being offered a different clinician.

Weeks later, another female psychologist, equipped with this understanding, made contact with Pria. She was able to develop a good therapeutic alliance, focusing initially on the "here-and-now" frustrations of treatment in hospital and relationships with the clinical team and family. This led, over time, to delving more deeply into her fears about her future, linking to difficulties in her internal world and arising from her past.

Knowledge, experience, and approach in psycho-oncology

There are limited training opportunities in psycho-oncology work beyond practical experience and very occasional training by established clinical teams. We have found that a significant part the clinical work requires "generic" skills that are not particular to a single discipline: careful listening, sense-making, and using empathy. There are unique skills and knowledge that are specific to teenage and young adult psycho-oncology, however, which we have attempted to share in this book. Familiarity with the various cancers affecting children, young people, and young adults is helpful, as is knowledge about a "typical" cancer journey and stages of treatment. Knowing about the various treatments and what they entail, their side effects, their impact and psychosocial toll, all seen within the context of the "adolescent process", is also important. We have experience of working with the dilemmas and conflicts around communication within families and with professionals, within which thinking about hope—with its retention and loss—plays a central role. An awareness of how the work can impact oncologists and psycho-oncology clinicians is valuable. We gain familiarity with the range of late effects that cancer survivors can experience and how to work with these. Facing mortality is typical, even with curable cancers, and the often profound, difficult, but enriching and humbling work of facing mortality plays a significant role.

Common themes emerge in our work. For example, young people struggle with feeling left behind by peers who progress through studies, complete exams, go off travelling, go to university, or start work, while the young person with cancer feels "knocked off their perch" and fears they will never catch up. A common difficulty in communication stems from the wish to protect or look after family-members, or from family members protecting their child from the cruel and frightening reality of cancer, and this carries the risk of the young person feeling entirely alone with their fears. Without the chance to share and talk about these, they may struggle to cope. Particular challenges, anxieties, and fears can emerge at particular stages of treatment, as detailed in the following vignettes.

Vignette 6. Familiarity with cancer treatments: Damian

Damian was an 8-year-old boy with cancer who required radio-isotope treatment. This involved being confined to a lead-lined room for up to a week after being administered the radioactive treatment—colloquially referred to as being "hot"—while waiting to excrete all the radioactive material. Being in proximity to him while "hot" causes radioactivity risk to others, so visitors and the clinical team need to minimize exposure and wear a Geiger counter to monitor exposure levels. A lead screen is placed between visitors/staff and the "hot" patient for protection. Items taken into the room—clothes, teddies, and so on—need to be disposed of afterwards. Young children and pregnant women should not come near at all. Damian's mother was pregnant during treatment, so she could not support him through treatment. Damian had an ADHD diagnosis, associated with hyperactivity, inattention, distractibility, and poor impulse control. He tended to run off when distressed or overwhelmed, to "walk off" frustrations. If he were to run out of his room while "hot", he would expose other children on the ward and the public to dangerous levels of radioactivity.

With our experience of this treatment, careful preparation could be made. Another family member that Damian enjoyed spending time with was identified. The reasoning behind this was explained in a way that he could understand. He was familiarized in advance with the room and staff. A play specialist spent time with him and his family, identifying and preparing a range of appealing activities and interests to occupy and comfort him across the range of moods he might have. A psychotherapist spent time thinking with him and his family about potential points of distress or frustration and how these could be recognized and responded to. A psychiatrist developed a step-wise escalation plan, which included behavioural, psychological, and pharmacological interventions, if needed, ensuring that Damian's ADHD was optimally controlled. A public health restraining order was identified and the process for implementing it established, so that, if all else failed, this could be used to protect the hospital and wider public. This preparation and the availability of a clear plan for patient, family, and staff effectively "contained" the associated anxiety. The treatment was given successfully, without incident. Damian left the ward cheerfully and asked, "What was all that fuss about?"

In some instances, specific difficulties will indicate the need for a particular evidence-based treatment, as shown in Vignette 7.

Vignette 7. Aligning symptoms to treatment-model: Penny

Penny was experiencing anticipatory anxiety and panic attacks prior to interventions or tests requiring needles. She was otherwise managing well and had a supportive, thoughtful family. Her mum was also terrified of needles, however. Penny was seen by a psychologist, together with a play specialist. A CBT approach was used, making links between thoughts, feelings, behaviours, and physiology. A combination of graded exposure, relaxation (breathing and progressive muscle relaxation), and modelling, with Penny and her mum together, supporting each other, allowed both to conquer their fears and Penny to become less phobic of needles.

In many instances, however, it is unclear which therapeutic approach is the best suited, and the evidence base is extremely limited. Interventions are reached by working tentatively, gauging responses, adapting, reflecting on the work and its benefits, and bringing in other colleagues or approaches when needed (see Vignettes 3, 4, 5). We find that input from each of the different disciplines and the range of professionals in the team, shared in case discussions, allows for more nuanced, insightful, versatile, and effective therapeutic work. By bringing cases to the team, different professionals take up a range of different perspectives and hypotheses, which are likely to align more accurately with those held by the patient, their family/friends, and the professional team. Sometimes the "formulation"—understanding of the factors that lead to difficulties— seems clear to the team, and there is a consensus over this. In other instances, it is less clear. The clinician must then manage and "contain" this uncertainty, exploring a variety of hypotheses and perspectives, holding these in mind, and testing them out, while remaining receptive, open, sensitive, and thoughtful with the patient. Sometimes a hypothesis or perspective is shared explicitly in a session, through naming feelings, thoughts, memories, or relationships and making links between these: an example is given in Vignette 8.

Vignette 8. Explicit use of interpretations and metaphor: Adi

Adi was a bright, forthright 12-year-old, the eldest of four siblings, of whom she was extremely fond. She developed a bone cancer and underwent painful surgery, radiotherapy, and chemotherapy. She struggled with physiotherapy and eventually refused this completely. When told how damaging this could be for recovery, she became angry and defensive. Adi had always been cheered up by visits from her siblings, but she became irritable and increasingly miserable after seeing them. She stopped eating and speaking, avoided eye contact, and became bed-bound.

She was seen by a psychologist, who encouraged her to speak about how she was feeling. Initially she was reticent, deflecting questions to her mum but irritably disagreeing with her responses. The psychologist suggested speaking to Adi alone and eventually enquired about visits from her siblings. She became more animated and complained about them jumping about and making too much noise, which gave her a headache. They were not careful enough and sometimes bumped into her, causing pain. She hated how they constantly wanted their mum's attention—they could be so childish. Suddenly Adi jumped and cried out in pain—causing the psychologist to jump too—complaining of a stabbing pain in the centre of her back. A nurse and doctor were called. The pain quickly subsided, with no cause found. On returning, the psychologist made a tentative link between what Adi had talked about and the sudden pain. They found a useful metaphor of being "stabbed in the back", recognizing the dual meaning of painful betrayal. Adi described her resentment of her siblings and their vitality and health, which sat starkly alongside her horrible, painful experiences. She was able to acknowledge her own guilt about this, and how—metaphorically—she might feel like "stabbing in the back" her siblings when they were able to jump, run, and laugh pain-free. She also recognized how they were having to manage without their mum—who was staying with Adi—and so were more possessive of their mum when visiting and less sympathetic towards Adi than usual. Adi began to speak about feeling so vulnerable, which she hated: as the eldest child, she had always been strong, capable, and able. She could not tolerate being "no good" at the physiotherapy exercises and experienced responses to this as undermining criticism. She seemed relieved to have understood and verbalized these feelings and agreed to the psychologist facilitating her speaking to mum and physiotherapist. They initially made visits from her siblings fewer and briefer, which enabled her to gradually enjoy their company again. Her morale lifted, her mood improved, and she made impressive strides with her physiotherapy rehabilitation.

Sometimes the perspective, hypothesis, or interpretation is not helpful when explicitly shared and must be introduced implicitly, the clinician holding the understanding or perspective in mind. Responses or lines of exploration become subtly influenced by this understanding, so the idea can be communicated gradually, in a more "digestible" and acceptable way, as illustrated in Vignette 9.

Vignette 9. Holding formulation and interpretations in mind; facing and not facing mortality: Bill

Bill was a young adult who was referred to the team after becoming overwhelmed with emotion on returning home following each cycle of chemotherapy. This first happened after a clinic appointment with his oncologist and his parents, where he had asked about the probability of his treatment not working and was shocked at the answer. Thereafter, he left clinic appointments whenever there were discussions about treatment progress, leaving his parents to act on his behalf. He was seen by a psychotherapist, with whom he engaged well. In therapy, there was an increasingly strong impression that Bill was gripped with fear that he would not survive and that his team would give up on his treatment. Repeated attempts to name and explore this with Bill were met with distress and subsequent silence, or with him terminating the session early.

The therapist brought the case to the team, feeling stuck, and she shared her own feelings of guilt and fear that she was causing Bill more harm than good. She wondered about the value of continuing therapy when this "elephant in the room" was so conspicuous and yet impossible to speak about. The team made links between the therapist's experience and Bill's fears about the oncology team giving up on him for being "a lost cause". Through his actions, Bill seemed to be letting professionals know he was not ready to face his mortality, and he experienced anyone introducing this as confrontational, cruel, and inflicting harm. This hypothesis was held in mind, and his therapist offered Bill the reassurance that she could see that "certain things" were too overwhelming, and so he would not have to think about these.

This freed up therapy, though Bill could still not speak about his fear of death, the sense that this would be "done to" him; he continued to leave oncology clinics early. A few weeks later, another patient he had befriended tragically died, and Bill spoke very movingly about this over subsequent therapy sessions. His therapist felt Bill spoke in reference to himself as well as to his lost friend, and she heard his comments as tacit contemplations about his own mortality. During the third such session, Bill's therapist felt grief-stricken and confronted by the emotional reality of Bill's death. Her eyes prickled with tears, and she had to work hard to contain herself from bursting out crying. Bill noticed this and voiced his surprise that she looked so upset. She spoke about the pain and sadness that she and others feel in loss, but that it need not feel dangerous or unmanageable when faced and shared. Bill became emotional too and was able to be sad with his therapist without leaving or shutting down.

At their next session, Bill thought they had been speaking about his death as well as his friend's. At last it became possible for them to work through this. He was able to verbalize his fears, including the damage this might do to his parents—especially his dad, who kept emotions to himself. A terrifying dream helped articulate a particular dread: in it, his parents lost interest when they learned he was dying, were not affected by the news, and quickly forgot about him after he died. Bill was helped to speak to his parents about these fears, which enabled these to be allayed. He regained hope and felt able to remain in his oncology clinic appointments.

Holding anxiety and risk within the team

Having the team behind us helps to "hold" the anxieties that arise from the uncertainties, which exist both in the patient and in the clinician. The work and the stories encountered can be very challenging, heart-wrenching, and catastrophic, confronting us with human vulnerability, pain, and loss. The support from and compassion towards each other in the team—towards patients and colleagues—helps all to face and process these and is invaluable. Clinicians receive weekly supervision and/or peer discussion with senior members of the team to help develop and manage the work. Informal clinical discussions with individual clinicians within and between disciplines also help to optimize therapeutic benefits. Equipped with the range of ideas and perspectives coming from the team, the clinician is more likely to arrive at an understanding that resonates with their patient. It also allows for safer work, by bringing "fresh eyes" and different views that protect from a narrow, singular perspective. Risks can also be considered from the combined experience and knowledge shared by the team, and in this way we practise more safely. An example of multidisciplinary risk-management is illustrated in Vignette 10.

Vignette 10. Holding anxiety and risks across the team: Dora

Dora was diagnosed with a haematological malignancy at the age of 15 years, and this was successfully treated. Tragically, she lost a number of family members to different cancers in the subsequent year. She became depressed and, aged 16 years, she made a suicide attempt. She received treatment from her local community CAMHS team. Unfortunately Dora relapsed two years after completing cancer treatment. She became despondent and pessimistic, believing she would not survive, having already been so unlucky. She was referred to the Psych-Oncology Team, and initially our role was to liaise with, update, coordinate, and maintain her existing treatment with the community team. After a particularly difficult course of treatment she told her nurse she felt suicidal, and an emergency psychiatric review was arranged. She was not felt to be at imminent risk, though she needed careful and frequent monitoring— both from the Psych-Oncology Team during treatment in hospital and from her local CAMHS team when at home. Over the course of the next three months she continued to see the Psych-Oncology psychologist weekly, but she needed periodic psychiatric reviews, especially when she felt overwhelmed. Her psychologist regularly brought sessions to the Psych-Oncology Team meeting and spoke to the psychiatrist whenever concerned, who, in turn, liaised with Dora's local CAMHS team when necessary. It became possible to pre-empt escalations without reaching crisis point. In this way, Dora's risks were held across the team, which felt reassuring for the psychologist, the medical and nursing team, and, most importantly, for Dora and her family.

Flexible working in Psych-Oncology

Over the years, our team have found that a great deal of flexibility is required to work with this patient group. Adhering rigidly to therapy models or treatments developed outside the arena of cancer is often incompatible with patients receiving cancer treatment, for various practical as well as psychological reasons. During treatment, the priority needs to be on the cancer treatment and on managing its effects. After cancer treatment, patients and families try to focus on re-engaging with "normal life" while managing clinical "late effects", ongoing clinical surveillance, and fears of recurrence, which can sometimes leave little time or space for psychological therapies. Some find the hospital itself laden with negative associations from their illness: terrifying fears, catastrophic news, gruelling and distressing symptoms or treatments, agonizing losses. A return to the physical setting where they had been treated, with those same sights, smells, and sounds, and the psychological "setting" of memories and associated feelings, can be a significant barrier, which needs to be crossed to receive treatment. Unfortunately, for some it is not always possible to cross this barrier, and they may not yet be ready or able to accept psychological support. Time, a change in circumstance, or a significant moment in life may be needed before they are ready to engage in treatment.

It is unusual to be able to offer the consistency and regularity of a specific setting, day, and time that is used in "conventional" psychodynamic psychotherapy, especially for inpatients receiving treatment within the hospital, but also for outpatients attending clinic appointments. Nor is there, in our acute hospital, the availability of rooms with one-way mirrors and adjoining rooms that would ideally support systemic family therapy. A psychiatrist can sometimes struggle to differentiate between the normal physical, psychological, and emotional repercussions of chemotherapy and a depressive episode, as in some ways these can present very similarly: low mood, negative cognitions, lack of energy, anhedonia, loss of appetite, poor attention and concentration, loss of libido, sleep interference. Few psychopharmacological trials exist to inform which medications are more effective and for how long treatments should be given. Benefits of treatments need to be weighed against potential side-effects in patients with significant physiological compromise. Effective psycho-oncology work requires therefore both experience and flexibility to recognize, allow for, and adjust to the hospital setting, these characteristic features of cancer treatment, and its aftermath.

A perennial issue is room availability, which is often unpredictable: changes may happen at the last minute due to infection-control or a room being needed for emergency treatment. Hospitals are busy, chaotic, unpredictable settings, often with scarce resources that are shared between teams, introducing a degree of competition between teams and clinicians. Appointments with patients in treatment need to be cancelled if a clinician/therapist has even a mild cough or cold, as the patients' immune systems are decimated by the treatment and a viral illness can be catastrophic. Systems for booking rooms, clinics, or organizing referrals often rely on individual administrators or clinicians, who may be transient or move between departments, leading to changes in these systems. Urgent scans or delays in treatment can interfere with timings of sessions. In most cases, the psychological therapy and assessments must work around the cancer treatment, scans, and the associated requirements for medical treatment. The other therapies—be they physical, occupational, psychological, dietician—have to fit around these. It is extremely challenging—and often impossible—to organize meeting with the whole family for therapy, when they are all struggling with both the practical and emotional tasks of looking after the family at home while also being available for their child in hospital for long and unpredictable periods of time. The toll of cancer treatment can be all-consuming for the family, timewise as well as emotionally. Indeed, at least one oncology consultant at our hospital advises parents to "put all family plans on hold and be prepared to postpone everything" over the course of treatment, as things are so unpredictable that events rarely fit with those plans.

The work done by the Psych-Oncology Team has been described using the analogy of a "field hospital" in a war zone: the clinician/therapist goes out to patients "equipped with a backpack" of psychotherapeutic tools. The treatment is delivered as and when it can be accepted and managed, when it is possible and safe to do so (R. Anderson, personal communication, 2013).

Work with the multidisciplinary oncology team

The MDT involved in treating children, teenagers, and young adults with cancer is large and diverse. It includes consultant oncologists and haematologists, junior doctors, nurses at all levels of seniority from healthcare assistants and trainees to CNSs, prescribing nurses, and nurse-consultants (Stark & Ferrari, 2018). Allied health professionals include physiotherapists, occupational therapists, dieticians, speech and language therapists. Play specialists engage with younger children and are essential for helping them to anticipate and tolerate treatments and procedures and to cope with prolonged admissions. There are activity coordinators for adolescents and young adults, who assist with anything from activities, sports, and distractions, to choosing a wig, mindfulness exercises, and psychological support. Social workers (Young Lives vs Cancer) are allocated to patients to offer practical, financial, and psychosocial support. Teachers and Connexions workers ensure that education is maintained where possible, liaise with schools, colleges, and universities, and try to protect patients' academic trajectories, employment, and progress. All these professionals meet in a weekly MDT meeting, where new referrals and complex cases are discussed to bring together the range of expertise and knowledge to optimize treatment. The Psych-Oncology Team, in addition to addressing psychological and psychiatric issues in patients and their families, also play a role in reflecting on psychological processes and dynamics within the MDT. By using observational skills, systemic thinking, and psychodynamic perspectives about conscious and unconscious processes within the MDT, the Psych-Oncology Team can help to uncover and respond to feelings and ideas that are generated when dealing with the sometimes very distressing and challenging cases and circumstances. At best, all these professionals work together cohesively to address the many different components of a patient's holistic treatment, which brings more effective treatment, and improves satisfaction for patient, staff, and clinical outcomes.

There are many pressures on the MDT that can compromise or interfere with the cohesiveness of team working. Some of these come from "outside": practical pressures, such as staffing shortages (which have become more acute since the COVID-19 pandemic) or insufficient beds. There is often competition for space, with pressures on room availability and other physical resources. Professionals also often compete for time, having to prioritize treatments or investigations, while also only having finite opportunities to offer their intervention during the day/week, especially when working part-time or covering multiple different teams.

Working clinically with young people with cancer can be difficult, emotive, and draining. Staff can find themselves deeply affected by the work, especially when a particular patient or family "touches" clinicians or "gets under the skin". This may be because of difficulties in a staff member's own life, because the young person or family somehow reminds them of—or connects with—a special person in their own lives. Some patients evoke, in staff, strong parental responses or an unusually powerful wish to care. The Psych-Oncology Team offers support to groups of staff, debriefs to process difficult or upsetting events, and gives individual support to staff who find themselves affected in their work.

Other pressures come from "within": for example, the despair from repeatedly delivering devastating news of such a serious diagnosis, or a poor prognosis, which can shatter a child or young person and their family's world, or the distress and horror of subjecting a child or young person to treatments that can be excruciating, and having to nurse them through this. There can be agonizing uncertainty about the future as treatment commences or ends, feelings of impotence, hopelessness, or guilt in the face of tragedy when treatments do not work or cause significant harm. When staff must support a young person and their family at the end of their foreshortened life, when the disease cannot be cured, this, too, can be difficult and painful. More positively, there is also the exhilaration and relief with successful treatments. This can sometimes lead to therapeutic "omnipotence" and unrealistic optimism. The MDT can become desensitized to the emotional reality of patients and their families, seeing cases day-in, day-out, while, for the family, it is a profoundly overwhelming and all-consuming singular personal experience. There may be minimization of the seriousness of a cancer that has an excellent prognosis, which the MDT might consider "good news" but which feels anything but that to the child who has the disease, and it can lead to an unhelpful mismatch of perception.

All these can "get into" the team or get between the team and their patients and interfere with the cohesiveness and integration of the MDT, as well as the ability of individual staff to function effectively. Sometimes these emerge as argumentativeness, hostility, or bullying within or between teams. There may be conflicts between individuals or between disciplines. Teams can become hopeless and nihilistic in the face of a series of bad outcomes. Or the team may begin to use defences, such as avoidance and denial—as individuals might in the face of overwhelming distress—so they become insensitive, make jokes, or overlook the seriousness of a situation. Individual staff and teams can begin to feel quite persecuted by a particularly difficult patient, family member, or situation, and may become uncharacteristically unsympathetic or hostile towards them. Unconscious dynamics within a family may be unwittingly "enacted" by the team, playing out dramas between team members that parallel the struggles within a troubled family (Britton, 1981). An example of this is given in Vignette 11.

Vignette 11. Re-enactment of problems in a family within the MDT: Pete

Pete was an adolescent admitted to the ward with an advanced cancer that was picked up late and was incurable. He and his parent had experienced adversity and trauma throughout Pete's childhood, including violence and emotional abuse. Pete had been taken into Local Authority care for periods in the past. His parent had significant difficulties that manifested in emotional instability, with explosive outbursts and very intrusive, upsetting, hostile behaviours when distressed. Although usually friendly, polite, and pleasant, the parent became aggressive and threatening towards staff when distressed, and had upset other patients. This generated concern, fear, consternation, and anger in staff. The Psych-Oncology Team met with Pete and his parent but struggled to engage them in therapeutic work. During an MDT meeting, staff complained about and criticized the parent, becoming increasingly intolerant of the unacceptable behaviour and its effect on others. Someone suggested the parent should be banned from the hospital. Another wanted parent and son to leave the hospital, believing that Pete's complaints of pain and nausea were exaggerated and he was simply avoiding being home with his parent.

They turned to members of the Psych-Oncology Team to demand they "sort out" the parent and were indignant at our "incompetence" at not preventing these episodes or implementing suitable consequences. The Psych-Oncology Team members felt impotent, attacked, and defensive. We brought to awareness the MDT's reactions, which paralleled Pete's parent's behaviour. We reflected upon the feelings of impotence, failure, and defensiveness evoked, which staff from the ward confirmed was how they felt when dealing with the parent. We recognized that these were very likely to be what Pete's parent found so intolerable and persecuting. Unable to engage with the parent's own failings and helplessness, it was staff who were experienced as cruelly failing Pete, and these feelings were, in turn, "pushed into" staff and, during the MDT meeting, into the Psych-Oncology Team.

The MDT came to understand that the behaviours could be understood as a process of communicating feelings that couldn't be put into words by Pete or his parent. In some instances, this understanding might helpfully be shared to allow a patient or parent to engage with these distressing thoughts and feelings. Pete's parent could not tolerate this, finding the experience of feeling understood only fleetingly helpful and quickly reverting to feeling persecuted and attacking. We, instead, focused efforts on helping staff to understand the processes in play and how to best contain Pete's and his parent's distress. Recognizing the need for firm but thoughtful responses to challenging behaviours, the Psych-Oncology Team helped staff to respond more constructively, sensitively, and in a less retaliatory way when setting boundaries. Although this didn't prevent all incidents, it did mitigate their frequency and severity. It allowed staff to respond to outbursts more effectively and to feel less offended and affected by them.

A crucial role of the Psych-Oncology Team is to notice and draw attention to these pressures, or misalignments. We can help to make sense of difficult dynamics that emerge in the team and to minimize the potential for these to interfere with optimal treatment and care. As well as attending to the individual needs of the patient and their family during the wider oncology MDT meetings, members of the Psych-Oncology Team also try to take a "meta-position", observing and attending to the various responses from the MDT. We try to notice when these feel inconsistent, distinct from usual, drawing attention to what is taking place and, where possible, making links between the feelings or ideas provoked and the reactions these have in staff or the MDT.

Conclusion

Scientific and epidemiological findings regarding cancer in adolescents and young adults have had an impact, and treatment of this vulnerable and important patient group has changed over time. With better recognition and understanding of the condition and how it manifests, services are beginning to address some of the broader impacts on young people with cancer. A Psych-Oncology team can play an important role in this, as it functions and evolves over time.

CHAPTER TWO

The cancer journey

Mike Groszmann

Pre-diagnosis

The difficulties we have come to observe tend to emerge at distinct points along the cancer "journey". Cancer often attracts metaphors of a journey, and one might assume that this journey begins at diagnosis. However, not infrequently a cancer diagnosis in teenagers and young adults comes after a long and protracted course of contact with health professionals. Reassurances are often given initially ("you are young, fit, and well"; "you worry too much"; "take some pain-killers and come back if it gets worse"), and symptoms or signs that might, in retrospect, seem unforgivably conspicuous are often misdiagnosed as the far more common aches, pains, lumps, bumps, and problems from which young people recover spontaneously (McCabe, 2018). A normal facet of adolescent development is that young people tend to feel somewhat invincible—in the prime of their life—and might themselves ignore or dismiss a symptom until it becomes impossible for them to function or it is noticed by someone else. Young people have greater physiological reserves and may not notice or may dismiss symptoms until the disease has progressed and become advanced. Because of these and other factors, TYAs tend to present with cancer later in the course of the disease than in other age groups and may become severely unwell before their illness is finally identified (Barr et al., 2016; Dommett, Redaniel, Stevens, Hamilton, &

DOI: 10.4324/9781003325475-3

Martin, 2013). Tragically, it is sometimes too late to cure them by the time of diagnosis, if the disease has already metastasized or progressed too far. We hear time and again of multiple attendances at GPs, paediatricians, or physicians and emergency departments before a definitive diagnosis is made (McCabe, 2018; Stark & Ferrari, 2018).

The beginning of the "journey", therefore, often precedes the diagnosis itself and is fraught with anxiety, uncertainty, and often with disbelief, which may be longstanding. Depending on the experience leading to diagnosis, trust for health professionals may be compromised from the start, especially where opportunities for earlier detection were missed or false reassurances were offered by unsuspecting professionals. From the outset, a scene may be set for shock, disappointment, fear, conflict, and mistrust. In these instances, the treating team face a considerable challenge in engaging and gaining the trust of a patient and their family, in the face of an often gruelling course of treatment ahead.

Diagnosis

The diagnosis itself can be a devastating blow for the child, teenager, or young adult, and for their family. Occasionally, the diagnosis might be experienced, paradoxically, as a relief when there has been uncertainty about symptoms or a dismissal of their significance by professionals or other people. Usually, though, it is experienced as a shocking injury. Cancer has particular, diverse meanings and significance for different people. Personal experiences often colour this—the miraculous survival of a relative who was not expected to, the death of a friend with a "treatable cancer", the agony of a loved one from increasingly unpleasant treatments: surprises, hope, hopelessness.

Culture—of the individual young person, their family, community, or country of origin—can also inform the meaning that a young person and their family assign to a cancer diagnosis. For some, there is a type of stigma associated with cancer that leads to secrecy and a sense of fear or shame. Cancer can be taboo in certain communities and cultures, or not to be spoken about in certain family cultures. For those, the diagnosis may be hidden; they pull out of their social circle and aim to get through treatment quietly, without anyone knowing. They may not even tell their immediate family or siblings—because of a wish to protect them from the worry, or from feelings of shame or denial and a fantasy that the less attention is paid, the more likely it will be that the cancer may disappear. A different individual, family, or social culture might take the opposite stance, seizing on the diagnosis and learning everything they can about it, informing everyone they know, "going public" on social media, and aligning with the various cancer charities, perhaps going on to fund-raise and champion the cause.

The moment of diagnosis is often associated with intense distress, yet coming to terms with the diagnosis and the treatment course is usually best managed by the oncology and nursing teams, and in most cases the distress resolves after a few days, once treatment commences. At that early stage, patients try to come to terms with their diagnosis and take in what the treatment plan will entail. Adjustment reactions are not uncommon at the point of diagnosis. This often manifests as fear and anxiety/panic, tearfulness, anger, denial, or withdrawal. These reactions to the diagnosis, while sometimes severe and disabling, are usually self-limiting. They come at a time of huge upheaval, as patients and their family meet a multitude of different health professionals and their days are filled with various scans, blood tests, assessments, and appointments. At a time when it can feel as though the world is crashing down, the young person and their family find their time filled with hospital visits. They meet their consultant, the medical team, and their allocated CNS. They are assigned a Young Lives vs Cancer social worker. They see pharmacists, physiotherapists, occupational therapists, dieticians, play specialists (for younger children), or activity coordinators (for teenagers and young adults), radiologists, and perhaps symptom control/palliative care teams. They meet professionals involved with delivering their particular treatment—radiotherapists and technicians, oncology nurses, surgeons, anaesthetists. They may see a clinician specializing in fertility, or various specialist medical teams, depending on the type or site of their cancer, or expected side effects of their treatments—orthopaedic surgeons, gastroenterologists, urologists/renal physicians, endocrinologists, cardiologists, microbiologists/infectious diseases physicians, and so on. Patients face new people, new places, new and often unnerving sights and experiences.

If a patient or family is not managing to engage with all this, they may be referred to Psych-Oncology to better understand the basis of this. We will work with them to try to enable them to attend the "work-up" to treatment. In practice, however, intervention at the point of diagnosis often risks adding yet more professionals and appointments to the already overwhelming timetable. Many young people and families simply do not have the time or space to fit in anything else. Others might not accept seeing a Psych-Oncology professional, feeling this to be manipulative, "tricking" them into compliance. Unless there are specific indications, psycho-oncology input is best introduced later in their journey.

Vignette 1. Adjustment reaction following diagnosis: Shinique

Shinique was diagnosed with a leukaemia and experienced severe anxiety and panic attacks after the diagnosis was explained and during preparations for chemotherapy. She was referred for psychological support. Multiple attempts were made to see her, but she was always busy with investigations or feeling too unwell to speak. The psychologist spoke, instead, to her nurses and the clinical nurse specialist working closely with her to offer suggestions and advice. About three weeks into treatment Shinique was finally seen by the psychologist, but she explained that she felt very well supported and had come round to the treatment. She no longer felt particularly anxious and didn't feel psychology was needed.

Commencing treatment

The very early adjustment difficulties are usually better managed by an experienced, sensitive, and ideally a psychologically minded oncology multidisciplinary team (MDT), rather than yet more new professionals being introduced (see Vignette 1). Sometimes, however, additional support is needed from the outset. Examples include patients who are so phobic or traumatized by the diagnosis that they cannot consent to and accept investigations or treatment. Some patients have pre-existing mental health difficulties that already require treatment, and close liaison and preparation is needed with the patient and their existing clinical teams (e.g., see chapter 1, Vignette 10). There may be pre-existing severe phobias of needles, swallowing tablets, hospitals, or entering scanners. Good play-specialists and activity coordinators are skilled at helping patients overcome phobias, but sometimes specialist psychotherapy is required (e.g., see chapter 1, Vignette 7). Others may acquire phobias after treatment has begun. Anticipatory and conditioned nausea/vomiting is not uncommon during chemotherapy treatment and can be extremely debilitating for the patient suffering this unpleasant symptom and become a potential disruption to the life-saving treatment being delivered. Interestingly, working with nausea and vomiting, which often become a conditioned "anticipatory" nausea and vomiting—developing nausea before chemotherapy, for example, triggered by the journey to, or sight of, the hospital—was a primary task for psychologists working in cancer care in the past, but with the advent of more effective anti-emetics, this work has become far less prominent (Kazak & Noll, 2015).

Work early in treatment frequently centres around improving communication between a patient, their family, and the treating teams. In the drive to begin treatment, a young person or their family may feel their concern or perspective is misunderstood or not taken seriously. We sometimes think of this as being in an "interpreter" role: taking time to listen carefully without the vested interest of encouraging them to comply with treatment, and then sharing this with the team. We may join meetings with the patient/family and clinical team to explain or "translate" the different perspectives and mediate when tensions or misunderstandings arise.

Vignette 2. Psych-Oncology in the role of "interpreter": Yusuf

Yusuf was a young adult who spoke sufficient English to communicate, though he was not fluent. His cancer treatment included oral steroids, but he became overwhelmed with distress when given these. He was referred for a presumed phobia of swallowing tablets. When seen by a psychologist, it was clear he didn't mind swallowing tablets, other than steroids. Yusuf described two family members who had had terrible problems when taking steroids for a different condition, and one had died from what he understood had been a direct consequence. Yusuf tried to discuss his reservations but felt these were dismissed by the team, so didn't try again. He agreed to the psychologist being present at the next ward round. His experience was explained, and it shocked the nurses and medical team. They organized an interpreter and had a medical consultation to better understand what had happened to his family members, and to better explain steroids. Yusuf felt reassured by this, and staff were more sensitive to his apprehension, which was quickly resolved.

During treatment

As treatment proceeds, the physical and psychological impact can start to take its toll. Patients may become malnourished, weak, and exhausted, which can impact significantly on their morale. Setbacks can occur in treatment, such as an infection (see Vignette 3), a blood clot that might lodge in the lungs or brain, or blood counts not returning to sufficient levels to safely proceed with treatment. These can trigger feelings of defeat, failure, and hopelessness. This state has been referred to as *"demoralization"*, as distinct from "anhedonic depression" or "clinical depression" (Kissane, 2017). Demoralization can leave patients and their families feeling hopeless and pessimistic. Clinical staff tend to adopt an optimistic, hopeful approach to "fix" this: "it will get better soon . . ."; "it's just a blip . . ."; "this is normal . . ."; "you just need more antibiotics . . .". This positive approach can help, but sometimes the response does not align with a patient's emotional experience and may be experienced as delegitimizing or dismissing. This can leave the patient feeling alone with their distress, misunderstood, and generally feeling worse. Acknowledging and naming the fears and feelings—"meeting your patient where they are at"—is usually experienced as more helpful than attempts to "fix" or counteract the loss of hope and sense of failure. Rather than disagreeing or attempting to convince them that their belief is incorrect, it can allow the young person or their family to feel understood and believed, and to have an experience of sharing the burden of their distress. This can make it at least feel more manageable, if not better. This approach—operating at the emotional (often irrational) level rather than just at the "objective" and rational—exemplifies the psycho-oncology approach. As distinct from (*anhedonic*) *depression* which can respond to antidepressant medication and/or psychological therapy and tends to improve gradually over days or weeks, *demoralization* does not respond to medication (Kissane, 2017) and can improve quite abruptly and completely—often following some good news or relief, or the experience of feeling understood and validated (psychotherapy).

Vignette 3. Demoralization in the face of medical complications: Sabina

Sabina was rushed to the intensive care unit after developing a disseminated fungal infection following chemotherapy. The infection caused jaundice and kidney failure. Despite antifungal treatment, her impoverished immune system could not effectively get rid of the infection. She could not proceed with chemotherapy, nor leave hospital for months, and she became despondent and miserable. She was referred for psychiatric consultation to consider antidepressants. The psychiatrist felt that this was a case more of demoralization than of depression and explained this. He acknowledged what a horrific, torturous experience she had endured and noted that she spoke as though her body were failing, letting her down, as well as her family and the treating team, and she would never recover. Sabina was struck by this candid recognition, which captured what was bothering her most and was not followed by the usual reassurances, which, she felt, were "false hopes". She agreed to meet him again. Sabina later explained: "Cancer is the easy bit—I wish I could just get on with that." Her mood picked up immediately and dramatically as soon as she was well enough to spend a weekend at home, which enabled her to regain hope and believe she could get through treatment.

Challenges at end of treatment

Psychological needs tend to vary with the course of the illness and the treatment programme. We find that some patients seen during treatment no longer need support once they complete treatment. Others, who managed well during treatment, will struggle most as they near completion, or afterwards.

We have found that facing the end of treatment is often another difficult point in the cancer journey. While some might look at this point with excitement and even exhilaration, we have found that this is often a complex, painful point that is fraught with uncertainties and contradictions. Some will experience the relief and joy of not needing further treatment or appreciate the feeling of being "released" from hospital, which is often the expectation after the long and difficult treatment period. Some paediatric and young people's cancer units have a celebratory bell on the ward that is rung to mark their leaving after the final cycle of treatment. Parents and families might speak excitedly about the anticipated celebration of that last round of chemotherapy, the final dose of radiotherapy, or the last hospital admission. It is not uncommon, however, for patients who were well psychologically during treatment to struggle as they approach the end of treatment. This may happen weeks, months, even years after finishing. Patients often fix their focus and resolve to "just getting through". The end of treatment can therefore be a point at which the enormity of what they have been through hits home. This can be extremely painful and overwhelming for some who have "remained strong" and determined throughout and finally let down their guard and allow themselves to contemplate what they had endured or what could have/nearly did happen. Some will be greatly affected by friends and acquaintances who are continuing treatment, or who relapsed, or who, tragically, did not survive treatment: so-called "survivor guilt" (Glaser, Knowles, & Damaskos, 2019; Perez & Greenzang, 2019). Some find the possibility of a relapse of their cancer in the future unbearable and are beset with "health anxiety": preoccupation and fear around sensations or pains that may herald a return of their disease. They may find, paradoxically, that they miss the reassurance and perceived safety of seeing doctors and nurses every day, of having regular blood tests and scans. Having spent weeks or months adjusting to the new routine of treatment, losing this may rekindle some of the fears and uncertainties experienced at diagnosis and in early treatment. Returning home without the clinical staff around may feel frightening and precarious after having had their reassuring presence, around the clock, for so long. During such an intense, formative time, close relationships are sometimes formed with staff—especially with the nurses, but also with doctors and other professionals who cared for them, and with the domestic staff, receptionists, porters, and others. These relationships can be very difficult to move on from, and doing so may trigger something of a "bereavement" that can add to the other difficult losses incurred by diagnosis and/or treatment. For a very few people, the uncertainty of the future post-treatment can feel even more daunting than the cancer and its treatment—so much so that patients have confided that they almost wish the cancer would return, bringing with it a level of certainty and a treatment regime that the post-treatment survivorship period lacks.

Many of the referrals to the Psych-Oncology Team are for patients who have completed treatment—some recently, others often months or years after treatment. For some, a life event, such as going to or completing university, getting engaged or married, a birth or bereavement, might trigger an emotional and psychological "storm" that reignites some of the worst memories, fears, and horrors of diagnosis and treatment. This may occur in patients who had not appeared to struggle during the treatment itself. Patients may have been well in the years between completing treatment and being "hit" by what they experienced. Others may have struggled but not felt ready or able to engage in treatment at that point, as described in Vignette 4 (see also Vignettes 1, 4, and 9 in chapter 1).

Vignette 4. Awaiting the "right time" to work on trauma after cancer: Annabelle

Annabelle, a 19-year-old female, was referred after she attended clinic for surveillance about a year after completing treatment. She could not stop crying through her appointment, though she could not identify what was so upsetting. She agreed to referral to the Psych-Oncology Team and attended the first assessment session, but she found that being back in hospital brought distress that she found embarrassing and confusing. She struggled through the appointment but could not face talking about her thoughts and could not access memories, either from the surveillance appointment or from her treatment. She asked her mum to cancel her subsequent Psych-Oncology appointments, explaining that she had been experiencing nightmares since returning to the hospital and couldn't even face the journey there, as it brought back the same feelings she had when travelling for treatment. She was not able to shift from this, despite discussions on the phone and written information about trauma, how it works, and ways to treat it. She preferred to explore what was available locally, and so her clinician wrote to her and her GP to summarize the assessment, inviting them to get in touch again if she felt ready to.

Soon after the second anniversary of completing treatment, Annabelle made contact and was seen again. She did not pursue psychological help locally, but her GP prescribed an antidepressant, which she took for six months. This may have helped a little, but she chose to stop a few weeks after her boyfriend had proposed to her, which helped her to feel more secure and assured. She described a nightmare in which she relived a particularly difficult moment from treatment when she felt dreadful, refused further treatment, and was sternly warned that she would not survive without it. She awoke with a start, feeling terrified, and recognized similarities to her experience during her hospital appointment a year previously. She began to recall snippets of specific experiences from treatment and link these to her current distress. Over subsequent appointments with a therapist, she came to understand that the return to the hospital brought back memories of moments during her treatment when she felt so unwell that she didn't believe she could continue. She vividly recalled the pain, sickness, and gripping terror of certainty that she would not survive, as she simply couldn't face more treatment but knew the disease would progress without it. Her oncologist's advice at the time, intended to be benevolent, took on in her "emotional memory" the character of a sinister, haunting threat: a cruel choice between further unbearable torture—further treatment—or certain death. With good symptom control over subsequent days, she had managed to proceed with treatment. She successfully blocked out details of this episode from her mind, focusing on completing treatment and returning to college. These "emotional memories" resurfaced at her surveillance appointment, though they were disconnected from her autobiographical memories, from which they originated. With her therapist, she was able to "process" these memories, creating a coherent narrative with the feelings and fears put into words, being able to share them, and finding relief in having these known and understood.

It is difficult to say what changed to ready Annabelle for therapy: the passing of time, further development and maturity, the stability of a relationship with her fiancée, a second anniversary of survival (anniversaries seem to be remarkably poignant and filled with meaning, even when they are not recognized consciously), or her choosing and seeking out therapy herself rather than her oncologist or family advising it? Perhaps it was a combination of all these factors. It highlights the importance of patience and working at your patients' pace, rather than what family or other professionals consider they should accept.

The team also work with other "late effects" (see chapter 6), where treatment is completed and a cure achieved but the patient does not *truly recover* and cannot move on with life. For some, the psychological burden of the diagnosis and treatment is so overwhelming, and the trauma of illness so great, that longstanding psychological adversity persists. This is particularly true in patients who had difficulties in childhood or a family that could not sufficiently contain their fears during treatment. Others are left with disabilities that range from the insignificant, to the inconvenient, to devastating. It may involve compromised memory and cognition, appearance, mobility, limb-function or limb loss, physiological function (e.g., cardiac, neurological, hormonal), or loss of sight or hearing. These may be temporary but might also persist for months, years, or, sometimes, lifelong. Whereas support—psychological and rehabilitative—is now far more widely available *during* cancer treatment, there is much, much less available once treatment ends. Young people may find themselves significantly disabled, but with very limited help, falling between the gaps in services that usually support people with disabilities and no longer having the cancer diagnosis that brings with it a range of help and interventions. Our patients have described to us how the sympathy, admiration, and allowances society often affords people going through cancer treatment can "run out" once the cancer is "cured" and treatment ends. Yet for some, this care, concern, and understanding is needed most as they attempt to return to life after cancer, most especially if living with disabilities resulting from the disease or its treatment. The expectation that people ought to "move on" and not dwell on their adversity—much as is experienced by people who have suffered bereavement—can leave them isolated and misunderstood.

Relapse or disease progression and palliation

Patients whose cancer has recurred, or another cancer developed after their initial treatment, may also need psycho-oncology input. Some find it helpful to meet with the clinician with whom they had worked previously, knowing that they have already established a therapeutic, trusting relationship, and not having to start from scratch. Others may feel strongly that they do not want to see someone they had previously met, perhaps because they now feel older and developmentally at a different point, or because that clinician is associated with the initial illness and perhaps the "failed" treatment. While we might attempt to gently question their decision, we have found that it is important to follow the patient's wishes about whom they see—even in instances when we feel they would benefit far more from seeing the same clinician they had seen previously—with the opportunity to question and work with this decision later.

While fortunately most of our patients end work with our team having recovered, we also work with young people who do not survive their illness. Sometimes our role is to offer a space to share the fears, sadness, anger and rage, regret, or despair that accompany facing a terminal illness, and/or to help communicate these to family or the wider clinical team. Sometimes the reality cannot be faced or accepted, and our role may be to help the young person, their family, and/or the clinical team to understand and make sense of this. While we do offer psychological bereavement support to families we have worked with and got to know well—it would be cruel to abruptly stop work with a family member at this great time of need—sadly our service is not commissioned to offer routine bereavement support to families. This represents another area of significant unmet need, with families relying on charity/"third-sector" bereavement support after losing their loved one. Our Trust offers an annual bereavement group event for families to remember, commemorate together, and help process their loss alongside other bereaved families.

Conclusion

A diagnosis of cancer and its subsequent treatment is a journey that no one would wish to take. An awareness of the distinct challenges at particular points in this journey can be important in helping young people and their families to navigate its perils as best they can. Being aware and prepared, accompanying the young person and their family, can make the unbearable somewhat more bearable.

CHAPTER THREE

Adolescents with cancer: a journey interrupted

Jane Elfer

A diagnosis of cancer during adolescence is rare, but cancer is also the most common cause of death from disease in the teenage and young adult population. Survival rates are better than for adult cancers, but the UK BRIGHTLIGHT study by Annie Herbert and colleagues (2018) demonstrated how 35% of adolescents visited their GP more than three times before they received a diagnosis. Their position between childhood and adulthood has also made treatment more problematic, as it is not always clear whether an adult or paediatric protocol is preferable.

I have been made aware, working alongside my medical colleagues, that treating adolescents is often more difficult because of these anomalies. It made me think about how adolescence is such a time of change, emotionally as well as physically, that it is as if treatments, physical and psychological, cannot keep up with this phenomenal rate of change. In psychological terms, of course, the young person in front of you may move from their adolescent self to a more infantile state of mind to an almost adult state many times within a session.

Adolescence is defined now as a period of growth and development spanning the ages of 12 years up to, and sometimes beyond, 25. As Flynn (2000) reminds us: "A normal transition through adolescence involves some measure of disturbance" (p. 68).

DOI: 10.4324/9781003325475-4

This *disturbance* can make working with adolescents more of a challenge, for they themselves may not know who they are or what they want, from one hour to the next. Flynn (2000) writes of the fluctuating states of mind in an adolescent:

> . . . one needs to remember that throughout adolescence, and indeed in any adolescent's day, there will be constant shifts backwards and forwards. [p. 77]

Flynn reminds us of the psychoanalytic concepts of primitive splitting, projection, and projective identification. These theories help psychotherapists and psychoanalysts understand the feelings engendered in them during a session with a patient, so that they can better understand the psychological state of that person. These mechanisms are ordinary, and everyone experiences them in everyday parlance. However, on a ward that is full of adolescents who have cancer and are frightened and angry, these feelings can have the power to make staff—nurses, doctors, or physiotherapists—also *feel* these emotions in a way that is unsettling, because they are not their own but *feel* as if they are. The "measure of disturbance" (Flynn, 2000) can thus be felt by all on the ward.

The ward may feel different with different groups of patients: sometimes more lively and typically adolescent, at others more difficult and dark, depending on how ill the patients are, how well supported by family, and so on. Adolescents may have a way of unconsciously splitting staff, seeing some as "good" and others as "bad"; it may be helpful for staff to think about this so as not to be placed in competition with each other.

Aldiss and colleagues (2019) published research priorities for young people with cancer in the influential *BMJ Open* journal. This group, which includes young people treated for cancer, places psychological support at the top of their priorities, alongside nine other factors, which include survivorship care and bereavement support. These three topics alone are huge and complex but acknowledge that most adolescents may think about life-and-death questions, but in a more existential way, if they are not facing a serious illness. Being diagnosed with a serious illness such as cancer pushes these topics forcefully into the mind.

The request for psychological support during or after treatment is not straightforward, however. As Aldiss and colleagues' (2019) research shows, psychological care is seen as a priority by young people, but the reality can be rather different. A desire for psychological support and acceptance of this may change rapidly from hour to hour or day to day. Many of our patients will say that they have no idea what to talk about;

they comment that it feels "weird" to sit with someone, particularly an adult, and talk about feelings. Where do you start?

In this chapter, I hope to give an outline of the different ways in which an adolescent may behave after such a shocking diagnosis. I write about how this can affect those of us who work in this area, and how all staff—doctors, nurses, play specialists, physiotherapists and occupational therapists, and others—can be involved in the psychological care of these patients. If we can withstand the challenge of working with this age group in a way that allows for growth in both patient and staff, the journey may be smoother and less complicated. It can also be wonderfully enlivening too!

I think for all patients there is a wish not to be a patient but to be seen for who they are. Adolescents are no different, and I am aware that at times this can be forgotten and that behaviours commonly seen among this age group suddenly can seem like a problem when they are in hospital.

Winnicott wrote in 1961: "The cure for adolescence belongs to the passage of time and to the gradual maturation processes" (p. 79). Our patients do not always have this luxury, but I hope that this chapter allows for a greater understanding of this challenging period in all our lives.

Diagnosis

The journey to diagnosis for an adolescent or young adult may have taken many visits to the GP and even to Accident and Emergency Departments. In January 2018, Herbert and colleagues looked at the timeliness of diagnosis. Pains in arms or legs will often be seen as growing pains or muscle strain from vigorous exercise. Fatigue and staying in bed until late in the day are normal states for an adolescent, so perhaps initially it does not appear that there is anything wrong. It is understandable that sometimes in the early stages no alarm bells ring for parents or for the adolescents themselves.

Of course these symptoms will often be down to a more ordinary cause, which makes the diagnosis of cancer even more shocking. Some adolescents, in particular, may sit as though they are untouched by such news, while their parents may be weeping. Talking with these young people later, I understand that the shock is so great that they are almost frozen, cut off from their emotions in a self-protective way. Others will immediately think that this is a death sentence. Often their experience of cancer is of a grandparent or even a parent who has had the disease. These reactions are not so very different from an adult response, but our patients may not have known anyone of their own age with cancer and so immediately feel very different from their peers. They may feel like a child again and turn to parents for solace or, indeed, they may reject the understandable concern and seem cut-off and hard.

Garland (2003) reminds us that the word "trauma" comes from the Greek word that is describing the breaking of the skin or, as Garland describes, "a breaking of the bodily envelope" (p. 9). I especially like this description for adolescents, as it seems to me to describe the way in which they can be absorbed in their own world, somehow concentrating on that huge task of growing up physically and emotionally. Cancer pierces that envelope in a way that is different from the other age groups. It can halt them in their tracks, isolate them from their peers, and disrupt that all-important task of becoming themselves.

I describe the event of a cancer diagnosis as traumatic because so often it is so sudden and unexpected. Even if the young person has been ill for some time, a diagnosis of cancer may still be a complete shock. Parents who might normally process more difficult news for their children are themselves often unable to function as they might normally in the early days of diagnosis. Staff may find themselves dealing with adults who are not behaving like parents but people who have become angry and sensitive, which can make everyday activities more difficult.

I recall the parents of an adolescent girl who was receiving chemotherapy for the first time raging at staff for not delivering it exactly on time, so that they could go home before the rush hour. They made complaints and appeared aggressive and critical, until a senior nurse sat down and listened to their demands. It became clear that the parents were so afraid and upset about their daughter's illness that they longed to just go home, where they believed they could "get back to normal". They accepted some psychological support and were then able to express their overwhelming terror and grief. This led to an improving relationship with staff and a cessation of the complaints.

The family is altered and affected from that moment of diagnosis. Their relationship with their child will change in that moment too. Adolescents who have been a source of conflict and concern will suddenly be placed in a different light. Guilt and anxiety about whether a symptom was missed or not admitted to by the adolescent may become an issue that stands between them. The adolescent who was moving away from the safety of home may suddenly find that they no longer wish to venture out. Sometimes it means a step back and a complete loss of independence and of confidence. They can no longer manage even their own personal care, returning to an infantile state.

Their newly acquired abilities to manage many everyday things such as travel and personal care disappears, and parents must rearrange jobs and their own personal lives to accommodate a dependent child again. A parent's freedom can disappear, and while this may not be resented, it can mean that there is little time for thinking or processing the trauma that has suddenly occurred in their lives.

Sometimes the young person may alter in character and become angry and difficult to understand. This vacillation between different states is not unusual, of course, in adolescents who are well, but I find it helpful to remind myself of what may just be ordinary adolescent behaviour and "disturbance".

Margot Waddell writes:

> ... the psychoanalytic picture is one that puts the emphasis on the complex relationship between internal states and external tasks; on *capacities* rather than *abilities*. . . . [Waddell, 2018, p. 15]

In the context of a young person with cancer, the ability of the young person may not have altered but, of course, they may not have the capacity to comprehend or process the diagnosis of cancer, and it can feel as if their secret, private life of fantasy and imagination has been revealed and may have been the cause.

I have met several young people, both boys and girls, diagnosed with a cancer involving their genitals, which has gone undiagnosed through shame and embarrassment. Sexual excitement and experimentation is, of course, perfectly normal and usually private, but the arrival of a tumour may lead to fears of having caused the growth due to masturbation, for example.

The sense of an attack on the self is particularly prevalent, as looks and appearance is all-important in this age group.

Jackie

I met a girl, Jackie, who was 17, just after her diagnosis of cancer, as she was inconsolable, and she, her mother, and staff felt it may help for her to talk with someone. She was crying as I entered the room on the adolescent ward. Her mother, who looked strained, said that she would go and have coffee and left immediately. I introduced myself and, before I could say much more, Jackie launched into a tirade of anger about her hair. Jackie explained that if she had known that she would lose her long, thick blond hair she would never have agreed to treatment.

She shouted at me "I would rather DIE than lose my hair!" I agreed. For a moment she stared at me, then continued to rage about not being given a choice and no one realizing how utterly devastating this would be for her. Once she had calmed a little, I said that it seemed very important that I understand that losing her hair was the most awful thing in the world for her. She could not even think about her diagnosis yet.

Jackie's distress and anger had been so powerful that her mother and staff felt almost as if they could not proceed. They endeavoured in a kind way to reassure her that her hair would grow back, that she would be given a wig that resembled her own hair, or that she wear any one of a number of fashionable hats and scarves. This only served to make Jackie angrier, and her mother and staff felt stuck.

It is unusual to receive a referral to the Psych-Oncology Team at this point, as generally it is important that the family acclimatize to this difficult news. They may all need to weep or rage, and to rush in with "psychological help" can make families feel that there is something amiss with their feelings of shock and horror.

Henry

I met a young man, Henry, on the first day of treatment by chance in the waiting area and sat quietly listening to him express his shock as he sat alone, waiting for the nurse to arrive to take him to the ward for his first chemotherapy. Henry's father returned, and I introduced myself to him. He looked rather shocked and angry and said to his son, "You've got cancer and now you've gone mad, too?" While I tried to explain what I did and that we were just talking as the patient was new to all of this, I had clearly disturbed this father.

I can only speculate on the reasons for this, but sometimes it seems as if the adolescent, full of potential, carries the hopes and dreams of their parents. A diagnosis of cancer can shatter those thoughts but also introduce a more vulnerable picture that does not fit with the media view of cancer treatment as a battle that requires strong, determined, and positive "soldiers".

A psychoanalytic concept is useful here: that of projection and projective identification. Melanie Klein (1946a, 1946b) is one of the psychoanalysts who wrote extensively on this human mechanism that we all use unconsciously, and sometimes consciously, to rid ourselves of uncomfortable feelings that are mostly uncomfortable but are, occasionally, the good feelings we have about our own attributes. I find this helpful to have in my mind when there are particular struggles with families on the wards or in day care. When a family seem to be especially combative or critical, it may be that this is how they are feeling about themselves. They may unconsciously be "projecting" all of their pain and anger into us as staff, who are so closely linked to their child's illness. While one could not say this to a parent, it may help us not to feel "got at" and enable us to see what might be done to ameliorate their difficulties.

It can also be hard for parents to believe that a son or daughter who, up until recently, was active, lively, demanding, obstructive, or oppositional is suddenly a patient with a life-threatening disease. This disbelief can easily turn to a sense of guilt for parents, and they will search their minds for things they may have done or not done that is the cause of the cancer. For some this guilt—which is, of course, unfounded—turns to a projection of blame. Thus if there is a delay in diagnosis or treatment, the feelings of guilt are firmly projected into the doctor or nurse who can unwittingly then feel blamed or to blame. These incidents are so important to recognize as they can easily set the tone for the relationship between staff and patient.

However, it can also mean that parents may blame each other and tension may develop or, indeed, they may blame themselves and lose their capacity for parenting, giving in to every whim and demand of their son or daughter. This, in turn, may make the young person feel that matters are much worse than they are being told, or it may mean that they feel less safe, as they are faced with parents who seem very different.

When a diagnosis of cancer is given to a young person, it is fair to say that everyone in the room suffers. This unbearable fact jolts a family from their familiar life and into another world, as described by Christopher Hitchens (2012):

> ...I see it as a very gentle and firm deportation, taking me from the country of the well across the stark frontier that marks off the land of malady. [p. 2]

Life for all the family the patient, parents, and siblings will change from this day. The processing of the news will come in phases, but initially there may be a collapse into grief, fury that the disease was not found earlier, or guilt that it had not been seen sooner. All of these emotions can be projected into attending staff, and it can be hard to remain able to think. As a nurse wrote to me in 2018,

> "... sometimes it can be hard to get anything right. I bring the medications too soon, too late; I am too sympathetic or not sympathetic enough. It can make you feel anxious about going into the patient's room."

To be present at such a life-changing moment in a family's life is breathtaking in an almost suffocating way. Doctor and nurses must do this on a weekly basis, and the projection of hope, trust, fury, or fear or one of the thousands of emotions felt in that time-stopped moment must land somewhere.

On occasion, if the family has a complex personal history or the adolescent has a history of psychological struggles, it may be helpful to introduce the service at diagnosis, to explain that support is there to work directly with the adolescent and their family or to communicate with the team in the community that has been offering that support. If, for example, the adolescent is linked to CAMHS, it may be helpful to get permission from the patient to contact the team, to see how best to support that adolescent at this time.

Treatment

The time between diagnosis and treatment varies according to the urgency of the cancer, but treatments such as radiotherapy may need particular scans necessary for planning and require masks to be made. The family may have time to adjust somewhat to this new world, learn some of the terminology, and form a link with their medical team.

The Psych-Oncology Team may not be involved with the patient in these early days, but we may be a part of the multidisciplinary team (MDT) discussion. This is a way of encompassing the patient and family to endeavour to make sure their needs are met. It may be that the family have a particular view of "psychological support" and firmly refuse any help, like the father mentioned above, but we may support the team or the member of staff with whom the young person has made a link. I accompanied an occupational therapist (OT) to her appointments with a young woman not because my presence had been requested, but because the situation was so painful that this member of staff was struggling. I "chatted" to the girl's mother while the OT worked with the patient, who was deprived of speech and lay moaning in a very distressed and distressing manner. Thus I had an experience of the difficult nature of these appointments and could offer support to the OT, whose interventions were vital.

Others, who perhaps do not have the advantage of support or the internal resources, may value more specialized support—if the young person has struggled with depression, for example, prior to the diagnosis.

Acting as an advocate for such adolescents may be helpful. I can recall a young woman who had been struggling with depression for some time and who presented as aggressive and attacking. When she was diagnosed, it was yet another blow to her already fragile state of mind. The Psych-Oncology Team were able to work with the nurses on the ward, who were, in effect, on the front line for her aggression. We suggested that, rather than offering a soft and gentle approach, they become more businesslike. This did not mean being cold and abrupt but, rather, speaking to the adult self of the young woman who appeared to be terrified of feeling like a baby, as it seemed to make her feel "as if" vulnerability would signal failure and weakness. We recommended using firm but gentle language and holding on to a protective line that the patient was not attacking the individual but the world for giving her cancer.

One young man, Ahmed, whom I worked with during his treatment behaved in a way that made his parents feel that they must apologise to staff for his rude and abrupt way of speaking not just to them as parents, but also sometimes to staff. Much later in his treatment, he was able to explain this as his terror of falling apart if he were to be more polite and sensitive to people, especially his parents. It would be like opening up the wound or stripping away the skin, a metaphor for the way that Ahmed emotionally protected himself, so that every encounter would be agony.

Wilfred Bion (1967) described the baby's terror when something unexpected happened as "nameless dread" (p. 116). This was a place of endless fear, as though the baby were falling into an abyss. One can recognize this in babies when they have become so distressed that they cannot find comfort even in a feed. It does eventually pass. This type of event is not something that only happens to babies who are not well cared for, but something that most infants will experience. It will remain tucked away in the back of the mind but can at times of stress be re-evoked.

A cancer diagnosis and treatment may cause adolescents to feel this sense of "nameless dread", so that they will resort to what Esther Bick (1968) called a "second skin". This is the equivalent of a coat of armour formed to protect the person from further hurt. Used in the way illustrated by my patient Ahmed during an especially difficult time, it is not harmful, but if this becomes a chosen way of functioning, it can prevent genuine relationships. Allowing space for a patient to express their imagined control of what is happening can allow space for a relationship with the therapist to grow, and for that part of the patient to be challenged.

It can help to make sure that the young person's space is protected, always knocking before going into their room or calling out over the curtain to see if it is okay to enter the bed space. As a psychological service, we need always to remember that this is, effectively, a patient's bedroom—somewhere we would not normally enter. In my early days of working in the service, I was over-zealous in my quest to support a very distressed, recently diagnosed adolescent who had been ambivalent about accepting psychological support. I returned to see this patient without permission a week after my first visit. My return was not helpful, and it was some time before the patient connected again with our service.

Some young people will need to have their anger heard in a straight-forward way. Rage that they will lose their hair is not unusual, for example, as appearance is so important to them. To offer an immediate solution, such as a wig, does not allow for the anger to be heard and felt but pushes it back to the young person. Hearing their upset can be painful, and the need to produce a solution can be tempting but does not allow the feelings to be really heard and taken in.

When an adolescent is diagnosed with cancer, the move towards independence is disrupted. Adolescents in the ordinary way will often vacillate between what can feel like a critical rejection of their parents and a desperate hanging on to them. Cancer means that parents will have moved back into close physical and emotional contact with their child. It may mean that that young person's development is disrupted to the point where they are too anxious to leave home, go back to school, or start work or university. At this age, body image is so important, as are friends—the "gang"—but suddenly all these are threatened.

Harold

Harold had been a studious young man when he was diagnosed with leukaemia. He was utterly shocked, and although he tried to maintain contact with school friends, he felt so fatigued by treatment that he began to withdraw from them.

He saw what they were doing on Facebook and, while their postings were meant to keep him up-to-date, to Harold they only served as a reminder of what they could do and he could not. He was afraid to see them, lest he show his frustration and anger.

He agreed to meet me after his CNS suggested he just "give it a try". She was concerned that now that he was moving into the maintenance period of his treatment, he would really struggle to attend school. Since this part of the treatment would last for two years, she felt this would be damaging educationally as well as socially.

Harold was thin, pale, tall, and gangly. His hair was slowly growing back, and he sat looking at me in the consultation room. I explained about the Psych-Oncology Team and how we worked. I spoke about us getting to know each other perhaps like a joint assessment. He was interested in this idea and we began to talk.

It is important when working with young people that they feel they have choice in whether to meet one of the team, and we would always ask that the patient agree to an appointment. It is not unusual for many of this age group to be reluctant to see someone from "psych", as most would rather avoid talks about feelings unless it is with their friends. These talks with friends do include a description of their feelings but may not include a way of thinking about how to manage them. Adolescents are known for their reluctance to talk, preferring activity (which can include a retreat to sleep), so sitting in a room with a psychotherapist can be a daunting thought!

While I might prefer to remain silent until my patient speaks and sets the agenda, this is often unhelpful for adolescents, as the intensity can be too much. They may react by not returning for further sessions. I aim to encourage the young person to feel comfortable enough to speak about what is foremost in their mind, and this may include some ordinary questions about friends and leisure activities.

End of treatment

The end of treatment is the time that has been longed for since diagnosis, but when it finally arrives, it brings with it the fear that we are no longer "fighting the cancer". Now comes the time of waiting for the next set of scans or blood tests. The vigilance of parents might increase at this point, while the young person may either become very withdrawn or the opposite, and begin to take risks.

One young woman drove so fast that she crashed her motorbike. While the motorbike was a write-off, she survived and reported to me how her friends were shocked by her lack of reaction: "I was fine, I love to drive fast." It was of some concern to me that she seemed not to care for herself or other road users. As we talked about this reckless behaviour, however, it became clear that she was convinced that her cancer would come back.

This is a very dangerous time for some young people, especially if they have to take certain medications to prevent infection or transplant rejection. I have known some young patients to die because they have refused to comply with medical instructions, feeling that there is no hope and so no point in taking the medication. This heart-breaking response may be because the adolescent omnipotence has been broken. They have a sense that their lives are already ruined by the impact of cancer, even if there are no external signs. The knowledge that their friends have continued with their lives unaffected by illness can make them feel forever different, and if their ego is too fragile, it may be almost impossible to prevent this "self-harming" activity.

Judd (2001) writes of a session with boy who had had a limb amputated:

> . . . he says his arm would never be the same again, and he would probably lose his right eye next. He feels he is on an inexorable path towards increasing impotence and destruction. [p. 57]

Allowing a space for these huge, life-changing fears to be spoken about is so important. The public view can be that there is a huge celebration to be had once treatment is over. The battle is won, and the soldier is victorious. But like any "battle", the landscape in which it took place will be damaged and will take time to recover. This can be one of the more difficult periods for patients. They are no longer actively "fighting" the cancer and being treated with strong drugs, and it can feel like standing still waiting for something to happen.

The trauma of the initial event can for a time be very present, so that a return to the hospital for follow-up appointments sparks absolute terror and sometimes days of anxiety prior to the visit. This can reduce over time but never goes completely.

Back to "normal life"

Returning to school or college, work or university can present some young people with a crisis in confidence. They feel different inside and often outside with scars, a limp, or a lost limb, or their body size has changed. It can be difficult to talk about their experiences, although often these memories are ever-present.

Margaret

One young woman, Margaret, described trying to talk to new acquaintances at university. She was asked what she had done in her "gap year". When she explained, some had fallen silent and others expressed sympathy, but overall she suddenly felt that a "gap" had formed between them. She did not want them to be full of sympathy, nor did she want their anxiety to "say the right thing", but at the same time she did not quite know what she wanted. It felt again as if she had now established some sort of barrier between them.

We were able to think about this and to try to find a way that left Margaret feeling more in control about how much she had to say to new acquaintances.

Some who have lost a limb cannot, of course, be quite so private, and finding a form of words for that young person to use can offer them a space to think about how much more they want to say about their experiences. Confirming with them that they have a choice about this can be very helpful. One young man made up a story about a motorbike accident, resulting in his leg having to be amputated. While I am not entirely happy with this line of explanation, I wondered if it allowed him some space to get to know people first before embarking on the truth.

Cancer is a more acceptable and understandable disease for adults, while for adolescents it can feel as if they have something that an "old person" gets: one girl described how she felt that her doctor was "weirded out" by her cancer, an especially rare form of the disease. This made her feel as if she was somehow at fault—that she must have done something to get such an unusual form of cancer.

While we are aware that young children will have a very active fantasy life, it may be forgotten that adolescents, too, will spend a great deal of time "dreaming" about life and relationships. Cancer may bring a very unwelcome cruelty to these dreams, and this will add to their lack of confidence. Those young people who spent a great deal of time on their appearance may be especially vulnerable, and there are a number of organizations that can help with make-up and hair. However, I have known young people who have continued to wear hats or headscarves for months and even years after treatment.

Nathan

One young man, Nathan, whose hair had been an important part of his identity had worn a "beanie" for years, which meant that he was unable to attend clubs with his friends and restricted him when he tried to get a Saturday job. Initially we had concentrated on the meaning of his hair loss rather than what it represented. Once we had moved to this, he was able to grieve its loss and then to reinvent himself as someone with no hair. This was a painful piece of work with many missed sessions, as grief involves much anger, too. Facing his friends in his new presentation was an enormous step for Nathan, but, of course, after the first two or three meetings, his friends no longer thought about his new look.

The temptation to always go for the positive aspects of end of treatment is understandable and important for some, but we need also to be aware of the loss of the young person as they were before treatment. Supporting them towards what is often termed post-traumatic growth is possible for some, but for others the grief is overwhelming, and we need to provide long-term support for these young people to move towards a life that is different from the one they had planned. This can take time and is only possible if a period of mourning has been allowed and supported.

Death

Stein et al. (2019) wrote in their *Lancet* series, "Communicating the diagnosis of a life-threatening condition to a child is not a single event" (p. 1161).

The news that the cancer diagnosis given to a young person has no cure, or that there is no further treatment, is a terrible thing for the medical team to have to deliver. It is, of course, even harder for the patient and parents. Stein and colleagues are, I think, speaking about the need for some families to have a more graduated approach to the idea that the young person may not survive. However, they also confirm, alongside many other studies, that honesty about a young person's situation is the most helpful. This is also true when a point has been reached where there is no further treatment to be offered. Telling the truth, though it is almost unbearably hard, is clearly better for the young person, as many studies have shown. In Sweden, Ulrika Kreicbergs and her colleagues tried to contact all parents whose child had died as a result of cancer (Kreicbergs, Valdimarsdottir, Onelov, Henter, & Steineck, 2004). Out of 561 parents, 449 responded, and, out of these, 429 stated whether or not they had spoken to their child about dying. The authors found that none of the 147 parents who had talked with their child regretted it, but of those who had not, about 27% regretted not having spoken about this.

I worked with a parent whose adolescent son was dying and who felt, after his death, that there were many moments when he had tentatively broached the subject of his impending death. She had found it utterly unbearable and had always avoided the conversation. It was an added source of deep distress in her grief, and I have since tried, with as much gentleness as possible, to encourage these important yet unimaginable goodbyes.

Each young person and their family will have their own way of approaching death. We can be on hand to support them if they wish for that help, but many do not and need to return home to be surrounded by family and friends in familiar surroundings. The staff members who have come to know the patient in hospital can feel a sense of loss at their leaving—or, indeed, a sense of relief that they will not have to witness that young person's death. It is important for staff to have a space to grieve, not as the parents and families will, but in a more ordinary, human way. The temptation to rush on, to avoid thinking about that loss, can be very tempting. However, making a space to talk about and express the sadness of the loss of life can allow professionals to continue with this vital but painful work.

Lanyado (1999) writes about working with traumatized children and the importance of a good work/life balance. She speaks of making sure that there is time to restore, enabling professionals working with these very ill children to continue to be present and to be alongside them and their families as they die.

There are times, of course, when we feel we are unable to reach out to the young person, as his or her parents feel that they do not want their son or daughter to know that they are dying. This presents the team with a huge dilemma.

Aydin

I recall a young patient, Aydin, whom I had known for about a year. He was 14 years old, and despite his very quiet nature, would ask for me to come and sit with him. At these times he liked me to talk to him. I had to try to understand how he was feeling by what I sensed as I sat by his bed. I would articulate my thoughts about what he might be feeling, and he would either nod or shake his head. He looked satisfied when I had judged his mood correctly, and it seemed to provide him with a way of putting words to his feelings without his needing to speak very much.

Sadly, after many months of treatment, the cancer continued to grow, and it was decided that further treatment was not going to cure Aydin or prolong his life. His parents were convinced he did not know and asked that no one tell him. They also made the decision to return to their country of origin.

On his final day on the ward, he asked to see me, and, filled with sadness, I went to his room. He was alone. I said that I had heard he was going home, and he nodded and looked directly at me. He said that he was having his PICC [peripherally inserted central catheter] line removed, and he looked scared. I said that the nurses would make sure it would not hurt, and he shook his head crossly at me. So I ventured, "You know why it is coming out?" He nodded vigorously, still looking at me, and I said that I was sorry. He burst into tears, and I put my arms around him as he cried. Then we sat quietly together, and I asked if he would like me to get his parents in, so that he could speak with them, but he shook his head. I asked if he did not want them to know that he knew, and he nodded again. I said that he loved them and wanted to protect them. He nodded.

It was a moment of deep sadness. I said that he needed me to know, and he nodded, and I said that he needed to know, too, that I would remember him, and he agreed.

At that moment Aydin's parents and other family members came back into the room. They bought cake to celebrate his leaving the ward. He looked at me once more and then turned and smiled at his parents.

There is not one right way to approach this painful subject, and we will all bring to it our own experiences and feelings. I do, however, always suggest that a gentle and slow approach is best, checking why the young person is asking about dying at that particular moment. Is it just a passing thought that wants some reassurance, or is it a genuine wish to know?

Conclusion

The aim of this chapter was to think about the impact of cancer on adolescents: to keep in our minds how this devastating illness can impact on this age group who, in ordinary times, might also challenge us and our way of working. I have worked in this hospital for many years now, and as I approach retirement, I feel a great sense of sadness. However, at the same time I feel deeply privileged to have worked with so many extraordinary children and young people.

I have, despite the often painful situations, found it to be among the most extraordinary and powerful work I have ever done. It seems strange to say that I have loved the work, but I have: working alongside all the different patients, their families, and the large MDT. Sometimes just being there to witness and hold the pain or sadness has been all that I could do, but I have felt privileged to be there to witness the journeys of these young people.

CHAPTER FOUR

Keeping young adults with cancer connected: a psychologist's reflections

Anna Galloway

Young adulthood and cancer

In 2013 NHS England published specifications for services designed for teenagers and young adults with cancer (NHSE, 2013). In this document they set out that 16–24 year olds had unique needs, both physiologically and emotionally. Before then, this group had been seemingly overlooked as unique in their own right. This led to delays in diagnosis, higher proportional mortality, and difficulties adjusting to "normal" life following treatment. With the development of these services, alongside the physical needs of the cohort, it was recognized that this group required specialist access to psychosocial support, from diagnosis to cure and beyond. These specifications highlighted the unique nature of this time point and a need for careful care coordination, thoughtful practice around decision making (with the inclusion of families), and specific attention to be paid to issues that are more likely to arise in young adulthood, like further education, employment, fertility, and pregnancy. It is within this context that, in 2013, I began my work in the psycho-oncology service, meeting young people referred for psychological support.

Illness as relational

Illness and death can never be isolated to the individual, each person is inextricably linked to a network of others who are, in turn, invariably

DOI: 10.4324/9781003325475-5

affected by that disease or loss. Illness is a human condition that we are subjected to from our earliest days. Simple childhood illnesses may be our first encounter: visiting GPs for coughs and colds, hospital visits for sprained ankles, time off school, and days in bed. Even these experiences are linked to an "other": whether that's a professional, a family member, or a comforting soft toy, we are from our earliest days linking our feeling unwell or being in pain with another. When a young person is diagnosed with cancer, the systems around them are also drawn in, consciously or otherwise.

The word "cancer" is highly loaded: possibly the most notorious of all diagnoses and one laden with connections to death and complex treatments. I have often been surprised by the age at which children will have heard and interpreted the word cancer (although not always accurately). I have worked with children as young as 6 years who have been able to talk to me about cancer and have developed beliefs surrounding it. They see adverts on television, know friends or family members who have been affected. I have yet to meet a young adult who has not been fully aware of the gravity of their cancer diagnosis. Even when the treatment path and prognosis is favourable from the outset, the association of cancer with death is often still present. For these young people, navigating this existential dilemma and confrontation with mortality, which is so uncommon in their cohort, can be extremely disruptive, not just for the individual but for the entire system who are forced to reconstruct their lives around it.

As a psychologist working predominantly from a systemic framework, I have found that, more than any other age group, systems and relationships appear to be particularly complex and abundant for young people. If adolescence requires "nurturance without the fuss" (Wolf, 1991, cited in Carter & McGoldrick, 1999) then what may young adults and their families require as they navigate cancer and possible death?

Here I present a number of clinical case examples of work I have done with young adults. I attempt to highlight the challenges, as well as the very unique time in life that interweaves with these young people's journeys. I am not attempting to provide an example of "perfect" work—indeed, never have my own boundaries, prejudices, and personal experiences been challenged more than with those I describe in this chapter. Although I do not reference all the theoretical underpinnings of my practice, I am heavily influenced by post-Milan systemic theorists and practitioners, as well as narrative therapy and the work of Michael White.

Creating a space for talking

Holding onto the notion of "well begun is half done" (Lang & McAdams, 1995, p. 78), I have worked hard to not rush into contacting the individual following a referral. I have found that careful consideration of questions such as "who is asking for what, from whom" (Fredman & Rapaport, 2010) slow me down and force me to consider what is really being asked for from a referral. While working in a TYA setting, I have often found that the young adults themselves (with their nurse or doctor) are the instigators of the referral to psycho-oncology, as opposed to younger teens, who seemed more likely to have had a parent seeking support for them on their behalf. This seemed even more likely for young people who had a particularly extensive disease or who had been told there were no more curative treatment options available. Taking time, where possible, to discuss referrals, contact the individual to ask them about their previous experience of help (Reder & Fredman, 1996), and consider the system as a whole has provided me with a context from which to begin talking. I have met a number of young people who walked into the therapy room and were unable to say what they were hoping for from therapy, despite having sought it. Never has developing a strong therapeutic relationship been so imperative in forming a foundation from which the subject of illness or death can be spoken about.

While working in paediatrics, I have often aimed to invite anyone who may be part of a "problem-solving" system to an initial outpatient appointment. Following an outpatient referral, I have found it useful to start together (with whole families or significant members of the system), and this has been vital with younger children, where the difficulties presented are often only resolved with the engagement of parents and child. Perhaps unsurprisingly, most 16–24-year-olds I have worked with chose to attend initial sessions alone, despite having been invited, prior to meeting, to ask along anyone they would find supportive or helpful. Despite the pull to offer family work, I am conscious of the need to offer a protected space to individuals if that is what they are seeking, and I find that relational thinking does not necessarily require multiple people in the room (Hedges, 2005).

Within an inpatient or day-care context, I have often been met with different scenarios and people in the room. More often than not, when a young person has been on the ward, they will have a family member with them. I have had experiences of family members swiftly leaving the room when I introduce myself; however, I often ask the young person if they'd like to meet alone, or for their relative or friend to stay. I have found that, rather than being a hindrance, having another presence can often offer a real resource to the talking we are doing. This has, at times, also included a nurse, particularly in an intensive care setting. This is, of course, dependent on the type of talking the young person is hoping for, and I am conscious of the pull to protect another from the very difficult things one may be feeling. Sometimes I will name this, if I'm curious that this is what may be happening in the room, which often opens up a frank conversation about whether to have someone join the conversation or not. What I have found to be particularly important about this setting and with this age group is the need to work dynamically, adapting to what is presented in the moment and not being too rigid with how you had been hoping to proceed, from one session to the next.

When working with young people, particularly those looking to talk about terminal illness or death, I have found that slowing down and giving the therapeutic relationship enough time to build is crucial. Often I have found that a good number of early sessions will be spent purely building rapport, identifying strengths and values, and understanding their networks and systems. Despite the current climate and with increasing caseloads and waiting lists, I see this not as wasted time but as essential to being able to create any meaningful change in work with these young people. The dynamic, of course, shifts when working with inpatients. The chance to grow a relationship more quickly is often possible due to the regularity with which one might be able to see them, the intimate nature of working at someone's bedside, and the chance of meeting friends and family members in the process. I have often found myself having very short, 20–30 minute sessions (often for practical reasons, such as interruptions for treatment or due to side effects of disease or treatments), but this has also allowed me to see them more often—perhaps twice a week—which I have found allows therapeutic momentum to build. Of course this is especially important if someone has been referred at the end of life, and the luxury of time is not available.

The diagnosis—co-creating how to live alongside cancer: Olivia

Olivia, aged 22, brought her mother Sarah to therapy. Framed as support being needed for Olivia to cope with her recent diagnosis of cancer, it was clear from our initial meeting that the "problem in focus" was indeed relational, as opposed to individual. For Olivia, she acknowledged her personal worry, the impact this diagnosis was going to have on her life, her job, her personal outlook—however, more pressing for her was how she was going to manage her mother's fear as she was going through treatment. Olivia's mother was cautious to express how she was feeling at first, keen to protect the time for her daughter; however, as the initial session continued, she did express her grave fear for her daughter, her own personal shock, and how she was now struggling to sleep. This dual processing that was happening was also leading to arguments between the two of them: Olivia would feel very angry at her mother for appearing visibly distressed during consultations and constantly checking on her daughter. Sarah felt frustrated by Olivia not telling her immediately if she was feeling unwell, and this was exacerbated by the fact that Olivia had not told her mother sooner about the symptoms and investigations she was having. They both agreed that, aside from the understandable upset and worry they were both feeling, arguing and tension between them was making the experience even more distressing. The focus of the work quickly became about how they were going to negotiate and co-create this new relationship, so that it would provide them both with what they needed.

During our initial sessions I was interested in how they saw one another and what they valued in each other. I learnt about Sarah's role as a mother, and how she had mothered when the children were younger. Sarah described herself as "strict but loving" and felt that it was important her children had boundaries. She was a working mother, working full-time when the children were younger, and she reflected on whether this was something she had wanted to do or whether it had been driven by the demands of the role. Interestingly, Olivia did not recall her mother being especially strict but, rather, as fun and loving. Olivia loved having her around and recalled weekends at home playing games together and having special days where the two of them would go out. As Olivia spoke about her mother like this, Sarah was visibly moved and joined in the retelling of joyful family anecdotes.

I asked about their more recent relationship, since Olivia had become a woman in her own right, with a career and a partner. They both described remaining close as they had naturally separated from one another. I was interested to understand how they managed conflict as two adults (rather than adult–child), and they described having similar conflictual styles, often speaking up and needing to be heard before being able to move forward. This need to be heard was a shared quality, and we wondered together if this in part was challenged when tensions arose between them in this new context. To understand the nature of the conflict, we spent a session tracking an episode (Hedges, 2005), which gave more information about the dynamics and communications at play during these times.

This renegotiating of a progression from a parent–child to an adult-to-adult relationship is particularly complex in the young adult period. Even simple decisions about who to be your next of kin, who will stay with you in hospital (if you want someone to stay with you), and how you perceive yourself (as child or adult in that moment) are more complex. Olivia had chosen to come to sessions with her mother as opposed to her partner of three years; however, for her this did not mean that this was how she envisaged the rest of the treatment period going. Sarah had hopes that she would be able to be alongside her daughter throughout the treatment—not being part of ward rounds, consulted on treatment, or being guaranteed involvement every step of the way was a challenge for her. Olivia felt certain that although she imagined wanting her mother with her at times, she also wanted to be able to maintain her adult self during this period and to include her partner. In this sharing of different needs and hopes it became apparent that clear boundaries were being constructed within the sessions through the talking that was happening.

Using the learning we had done in previous sessions about roles within their family and what they appreciated in one another, we were able to elicit the times that would be most vital for togetherness to be happening. Olivia's appreciation of her mother's comfort during periods of fear helped us to understand that if there were to be times of feeling very unwell or before important results, Olivia would want her mother there. Sarah was able to acknowledge the need for Olivia's personal autonomy and choice in who she shared different parts of her journey with. We considered who may be able to act as a confidant to Sarah at periods of worry or stress, as Olivia did not feel it could be her mother at such times. We broadened the system from beyond the two of them in the room and mapped out who else was available and present and could act as a resource during this time.

Our final session came after three months, having seen each other roughly fortnightly and sometimes less. Olivia was having treatment; she had required two inpatient stays, and on those occasions had asked for her mother to stay with her, which Sarah was happy to do. Olivia had maintained her relationship with her partner, returning between stays to live at their shared flat rather than at her parents' home, which had been an expectation of her mother early on. Tension between mother and daughter appeared significantly reduced, and explicit conversations about what was going to happen allowed Sarah to feel confident things were not being hidden from her and also helped Olivia to feel that she was being respected as an adult. What we did not resolve was "worry", nor did we prevent periods of sadness, loss, and distress; however, creating a safe framework around this unchartered world allowed for that to be cushioned somewhat.

Cancer-free—reclaiming identity: Josh

Josh was a 20-year-old university student living in London. He had just finished treatment for testicular cancer and had been referred for psychological support by his consultant, who felt he was appearing "flat" and "subdued" in their recent consultation. Josh attended the appointment alone.

Our first session was spent predominantly getting to know Josh: who he was, what he did, what interested him. I heard about his family—supportive parents, a younger brother, and some friends who he was very close to. When asked, Josh tentatively offered me the story of when he had first noticed a lump. He appeared nervous about mentioning this, and I was aware of the dynamic of being with a stranger of the opposite sex and how he might be able to find a language for talking about this with me. Sadly for Josh, his reticence about seeking help for this lump meant that he did not tell anyone for a number of months, only eventually letting his father know, and then being supported to go to the GP. Josh worried this meant that treatment had needed to be more extensive than it might have been, and he was aware that this had also had a significant effect on his parents, who were devastated that he hadn't spoken earlier. I wondered if this was something he wanted to speak about in our sessions, as it was a dominant part of his narrative in that first meeting. However, Josh, was now cancer-free, and he wanted to look forward and think about the future.

Our next few sessions following this initial one were spent thinking about how to get life "back on track": how would Josh know he'd reached where he was hoping to, what steps did he think this would take, how might his values and world view be interwoven and privileged by his new outlook on life. Josh spoke thoughtfully about this and engaged well in these conversations, but we appeared to be making slow progress, and I wondered what Josh was hoping for before he would feel he had got what he wanted out of our sessions. I had hypothesized from the outset that the effect of having one testicle may require some psychological adjustment for a young single man; however, he had not brought this, and something had stopped me from testing this hypothesis in sessions with him. I questioned myself in supervision about whether this was due to a silent withholding of permission from Josh, or a reticence and self-consciousness from me. After four sessions I felt work had stalled, and so I asked: "and what effect is the treatment and surgery to your testicle going to have on moving this plan forward?"

Rather than shutting this conversation down, Josh appeared to be visibly relieved by me asking this question directly, and I felt frustrated I hadn't asked this earlier, although I wonder if our relationship needed to be established before being able to begin this more intimate talking. Josh let me know he was fearful about what this might mean for future children, but, more strikingly, how he was meant to move forward with sexual relationships: should he tell people beforehand, should he declare it before getting into a relationship, does this make him seem less masculine to women? For Josh, as a young man who had been made to step out of life as he knew it before, being able to begin having sexual relationships again was a very important factor in moving on with his life. He felt that being able to venture into the world of relationships and dating would be a marker for him of the return of normality.

Josh let me know that this was particularly significant at this point, due to his perceived infantilization during treatment. He spoke about what he described as his move from "almost independence" to "total dependence" on his parents for all aspects of his life. When he was first diagnosed, he had consciously chosen to stay in his shared flat in London with his friends; however he had been shocked by how quickly life had changed and, following surgery, chose to move back to his parents' house in Oxfordshire. He said this was his decision, but in reality he felt there was no choice in it. He subsequently described a stripping of his preferred identity, the loss of who he was, and the sense of vulnerability that came with this. He was reliant on his parents for lifts to and from hospital. When he had admissions, one of them would sleep in the room with him, which he had wanted but which also reminded him of his sense of regression. He would have physical examinations of his testes, and although parents would step out or look away, Josh was acutely aware of their knowledge of this act and a self-consciousness that this brought. At his sickest, during chemotherapy, Josh required help going to the toilet, having a shower, and dressing—when possible, he preferred this to be a parent rather than a nurse, who were often female and not far from his own age. His loss of all bodily hair also contributed to the child-like identity he felt had become dominant. I asked Josh if he felt his parents would have felt this shift in their relationship, and he said he believed they would have.

It felt important for us to give time to hearing about this stripping back of identity. However, throughout this telling, I tried hard to listen for responses or "acts of resistance" to this trauma (Wade, 1997) that would highlight exceptions to the rule and semblances of that preferred identity. As Josh spoke about the sense of total dependency on another, I was curious to understand how he had made it known to others what it was he needed of them. He told me that even at his lowest points he felt able to say "no" when he needed to: no to the nurses he felt embarrassed around, no to his parents leaving when he was particularly afraid or fatigued, no to staff when he kept getting interrupted and needed to sleep. The ability to say no, to assert his needs at that point, regardless of what the need was, represented acts of assertion, independence and self-knowledge that Josh was able to hold onto.

During our remaining sessions we worked hard to recognize together those small acts of resistance, of defiance, that Josh recognized as himself (pre-cancer). To do this, I needed to attend to some of the smallest details in the narratives I was given, in the stories Josh told, and, rather than always offering them to him, helping him notice alternative narratives in a bid to thicken his preferred identity. We slowly moved back to the initial questions of talking with people and potential partners about his experience, but this time from a position that felt much stronger, safer, and enduring. Josh was able to think about possible options for such talking, whether there was a need for him to "declare" it to all women he met (which, he felt, was not needed), and he decided that he would only speak with a potential partner about it if he thought the relationship might have a future. Instead, he would allow himself to be the carefree, assertive, independent man he was and give himself permission to trust his instincts—something that had got him through some of the most traumatic and challenging times he had experienced.

When cure is not possible: talking with young people about death and dying

So what happens when a young person is told that there is no cure for their disease? Even for those with very treatable conditions, the initial diagnosis often brings with it a recognition of one's mortality. Fear of death or fear of the future is very common during this time. When a young adult is told that there will be no cure, how do they begin to comprehend and make sense of their lost future? It is often at these times that communication is especially difficult. How do we begin to speak about something so unspeakable?

As young people and families struggle to speak about their loss, fear, and sorrow following a terminal diagnosis, treating teams can also find communication getting harder. Even for very experienced medics, nurses, and other members of the multidisciplinary team (including psychologists), it can still be extremely challenging to talk to young people and their families about death. Various factors can contribute to this, including relationships based on hope having already formed with the patient during treatment, personal experiences of loss, how we may identify with that patient, and many, many more. If we find it challenging, how, then, can a young person or family member find the words to talk about it?

A significant proportion of the work I have done with young adults has been with those who have a poor prognosis or an incurable disease, or are at end of life. I have found that sometimes this confrontation with mortality has been the springboard for requesting (or agreeing to) psychological support. Of course, learning of your premature death is likely to trigger distress and despair at any age, I have often wondered if this period of transition, of future focus and aspiration, leads to an even more profound impact on self, identity, and relationships. At times I have also found it to be extremely demanding, personally, to support these young people as they navigate such burdens, as I, too, would prefer to sustain society's illusion that young people do not die.

A first experience of (not) talking: Rachel

I first worked in a medical context as a second-year trainee clinical psychologist with adults with respiratory conditions. I remember on my first day of placement being invited to meet with Rachel, who had just turned 18, was very unwell, and was expected to die within the next few months. She had been referred by her consultant because she had stopped talking to the team and seemed very "angry". As an eager trainee psychologist I went to her hospital room unannounced, hoping she would be willing to talk to me. In hindsight, this now seems absurd—why would she be willing to talk to this complete stranger introducing herself as a trainee psychologist, if she was not speaking with anyone? I was met, unsurprisingly, with silence but not total rejection, so I diligently kept returning for 10-minute bursts. Over the weeks we had some exchange, though often the only thing she would talk about was her family and what they were doing.

As she became more unwell over the weeks, the "elephant in the room" became more and more apparent. I couldn't find the words to verbalize what that was, and she, too, never mentioned the unmentionable, although often during that time I wondered to myself if the silence was speaking. Sadly, Rachel died a few weeks after we had begun meeting—what if I had been able to speak about death? Should I have talked about it? Did she want to, or absolutely not? Is it enough to speak around it, or is that silencing?

This first professional experience of death taught me to slow down, reflect on my own position, and roll with the work, adapting, being flexible, and sometimes needing to be brave. I have also found that, at times, this work requires more than one psychologist (when working with multiple people). It often requires time for reflection and discussion, and sometimes in that moment, for personal reasons, it is not possible at all. Principally, knowing the difference is what matters.

Staying connected—speaking about the unspeakable when cure is not possible: Lyra

Lyra was a 19-year-old woman. She had been diagnosed with a very rare cancer, which was already wide-spread at diagnosis and where treatment options were offered but with no curative intent. Her disease was currently being managed with a medication intended to slow down the progression. At the point of diagnosis she was feeling well, she was not being treated with chemotherapy, which had previously made her feel very ill, and she had a lot of energy.

Lyra had let me know clearly in our earlier "relationship to help" conversations that she was reticent about speaking to a psychologist, only agreeing to give it a go because she felt alone with her fears. She had not had any previous psychological support, despite being offered it from the point of diagnosis, but had found the emotional support provided by her clinical nurse specialist (CNS) useful. She had relied heavily on support from her CNS before appointments or important scans, seeking reassurance and comfort from her rather than from family members.

I met with Lyra for an initial session, which she came to alone. In that session I heard about her life outside hospital, attending college, meeting with friends, shopping, going to parties, watching films. She let me know about some of the people in her life, including her best friend and sister. I was curious to hear more about who lives at home with her, and she said that she also lives with her mother and younger brother. When asked about her father, she said he had died when she was a child, also of cancer and that she was from a large Italian family, her father being Italian and her mother from the United Kingdom. She told me about some of the customs they still hold onto in the family, despite her father no longer being alive, and about her father's family, who live in Italy, and their visits to the United Kingdom every few years.

I wondered why Lyra had decided to meet with a psychologist now. I heard that she had recently been given some bad news regarding her cancer progression, and this had triggered increased feelings of anxiety and fear. She spoke about having lived with the knowledge that her condition wasn't going to be cured ever since initial diagnosis, and the challenges that had brought with it. These included worrying about starting new relationships, in particular romantic relationships (feeling that it would be unfair on "the other"), wanting to carry on with everything important to her, such as college, although the uncertainty of not knowing how long she may have left loomed heavy. What was most difficult for her, however, was the impact of this most recent progression in her disease on her family and on their ability to communicate with one another. It was impossible to speak about the future, and it was impossible to speak about the now. Speaking about anything had stopped.

I was interested to hear more about her values and what was particularly important to her about being able to talk about the future with those she loved. I asked more about how talking had worked in her family up to this point. She said that they had always been very close; she had been able to speak to her mother about things other teenage girls may not be able to, such as relationships and sex. They would debate different issues around the table; with Lyra often taking the lead. Her father had been a dynamic figure. He'd had a thick Italian accent and would move between languages without a thought and at great speed. She remembered how quiet the house had seemed after he had died, and now this most recent silence was deafening.

Many of our early sessions were spent "talking about talking" (Fredman, 1997). I felt this was useful to learn more about how communication worked within their family: for example, who Lyra would speak with about worries or fears. How would she know when it was or wasn't possible to talk? How do different members of her family use talking? This knowledge offered me a template of how communication and connectedness worked when times were simpler. Until this point Grace, her sister, had been someone she felt she could speak to about her diagnosis. She valued Grace's quiet nature, her ability to listen and not necessarily respond with an answer. She said she wasn't looking for people to give her answers but, rather, to show they had heard what she was saying. Her mother had been someone who she could talk to; however, she was more wary about speaking to her mother about the more distressing elements of her diagnosis and treatment. She preferred to protect her mother as much as possible and felt she had been through enough already. Lyra and her brother talked about different things—she appreciated his humour and ability to change the subject when people were becoming upset. Their more "serious" talking happened at times when they were in the car together or doing something more practical.

We spoke about the silence. I asked her to describe this to me. She had invited her mother into the consultation with her when she was given the information that her cancer had started to progress further, and therefore the treatment that had previously been working had now stopped being effective. Lyra did not feel this came as a surprise to her; she said that she knew somehow that this would be the outcome, although it did, of course, cause her great distress. Her mother had responded to the information with a lot of questions, queries about specialists, and the response that it will be ok. Lyra felt that her mother was coping with the information that she had been given by pretending it wasn't happening. I wondered whether this was a helpful approach for Lyra or not: she thought it might be for her mum, but that it meant they were no longer speaking at all, because they were on such different pages.

We met weekly. Lyra was going to college not far from the hospital and was keen to come regularly. During our sessions together we explored these ideas: what Lyra might want things to look like with her family, and how we might go about making small changes. Together we came up with small challenges to try and bring forth the connections in the family, which were fused together with their joint values and histories. For example, one week Lyra's challenge was to find a time to sit with her sister and talk to her about her exams, and she was challenged to ask her mother about mundane tasks, such as who was going to do the washing. Even these totally unrelated conversations allowed some noise to come back into the house. When Lyra felt she had practised talking with me—speaking frankly about her fears, her concerns for her family after her death, and fears of what death might be like, we considered what her main hope was for her life now. What was most central for Lyra was to have her family back: the laughter, the intimacy, the connectedness. For that, we needed them in the room.

Lyra invited her family into the sessions, and I invited another colleague to act as a "team" for systemically informed family work. This part of the work felt extremely important to me. However, because I had already developed a strong therapeutic relationship with Lyra, it placed me in an unusual position as a lead therapist. I knew Lyra very well, I knew her fears as well as her thoughts about her family. I knew things about her family they were unlikely to know I knew. When trying to hold a position of curiosity with everyone in the room, I had to be conscious of my pre-existing hypotheses as well as my beliefs and thoughts about what might happen. I was grateful when a psychologist colleague was able to join and act as my team, holding in mind the positions of everyone in the room, challenging my sometimes leading questions, and working with me to offer in-room reflections.

Reflecting with another in the room in front of the family appeared to be the greatest tool in offering a shift in the dynamics at play. During our first family sessions hearing everyone's hopes for the meeting and asking future-focused questions helped steer our talking. However, unsurprisingly, no one raised Lyra's condition and prognosis as a factor requiring attention. Rather, agenda items included worry around more arguments happening at home, different people not doing delegated tasks in the house, and frustrations about how people were talking to each other.

After two sessions of feeling like we were talking in circles about people's dissatisfactions with one another, my colleague and I asked the family to take a listening position, while we shared our reflections and our hypotheses about what we might be missing in the room. In one of these conversations my colleague reflected the themes that were emerging and the common factor between them, which was how people were talking with one another, rather than the content of what was being said. I wondered if, indeed, we were missing something that felt harder to talk about. I considered not explicitly mentioning Lyra's health, which felt the more comfortable option in the room; however, I decided to name it to my colleague. "I'm curious to understand if one of the things affecting talking at the moment is the recent news Lyra received about her cancer?" I knew this was likely to be difficult to listen to, but, equally, I wanted to offer a space for this if the family wanted to take this up—which they did. On turning back to the family following our reflections, each one was able to speak thoughtfully about their worry about talking about cancer.

We found that the subsequent three family sessions were far more fruitful, and changes in how they were interacting with one another were clear. We reflected together how we hoped this talking might be able to continue following our sessions, how distress can be shared, how it can be tolerated alongside happiness and laughter. We spoke about "hope", which had become a hidden feeling in the family—almost a taboo, representing denial. In our talking this shifted, and the family were able to see "hope" as a valuable tool in coping with what was happening. We used "re-membering conversations" (White, 1988) to bring Lyra's dad into the room, which offered great resource and strength, as well as reflections on how they coped as a unit when he died and leading up to his death.

Although I was more than happy to continue meeting with Lyra for ongoing individual support when the family sessions came to an end, the frequency of these reduced greatly, and mainly occurred when she was having a period of feeling especially anxious. The connections that were highlighted and strengthened through the sharing of values, skills, and love with her family were by far the most valuable aspect of the work. Lyra lived for another year after these sessions, she told me about the power of her family network in allowing her to keep living despite knowing she was dying. For Lyra, relationships were the sole reason for her to keep living, and her ongoing connection to her father despite his death offered her comfort as she neared the end of her life. When Lyra died, I felt deeply moved and the connection I had made to her did not dissipate following her death. I can still clearly recall many of our conversations, and these help inform my work today; for me this is my way of honouring her legacy.

Re-connecting when death is imminent: Priya

I first met Priya on the ward when she had been told her tumour was growing too rapidly to be operated on. Due to the location of the tumour this meant she had short weeks left to live. Priya had asked to speak to someone who had not been involved in her care up to this point. She had a very strong relationship with her CNS due to her extensive cancer journey and until this point had declined psychological support. I heard from her CNS that Priya seemed "flat, detached, and unwilling to speak about her disease".

I was keen to start building trust and rapport from the onset of our work. I prefaced our first meeting by letting her know we did not need to speak about anything she didn't want to, and that I would be led by her. We spent our first session quietly speaking at her bedside (as she was in a bay). I learnt about her family and friends, life before cancer, her skills, values, and dreams. She came alive when speaking about her friends, her best friend and what she was doing, how they made each other laugh. She valued friendship, family, and trust. Her parents had both been born and raised in India; she talked to me about the traditions and customs they still enjoyed as a family and her favourite foods. Although she didn't identify as religious, she found comfort in knowing her parents both followed their faith closely. Narrative approaches informed my questioning as I looked to thicken her preferred identity, one that had been subjugated by her diagnosis and recent information.

We agreed to meet regularly, and I aimed to see her as an inpatient twice weekly where possible. I was able to start asking more questions about talking and how it worked in her family (Fredman, 1997): who spoke with whom, how they spoke about challenging situations, what effect talking had on different members of the family. I learnt that, generally, they had been an open family, people that she could talk to if something had gone wrong in school or when she was having a difficulty. She has found speaking with her mother a great help at times of stress, finding it cathartic and also valuing her mother's ability to find solutions that she hadn't thought about. I asked her about how talking worked when she was first diagnosed with cancer. Priya had been able to talk to her parents, who were extremely anxious but didn't hide it from her. She said she preferred this and did not want them to try to protect her. It had allowed her to express her own anxiety.

I asked how talking was going at the moment. She told me that talking had stopped since her meeting with her consultant just over a week ago, and hearing that they would not operate again and that therefore she did not have long to live. Her parents were asking her questions about whether she was eating or if she needed anything, but there were no tears or long conversations about their worries. I offered a hypothesis: "I wonder if talking has become too difficult since that meeting, and therefore it's not happening at all." She agreed with this. At this point she told me that there was nothing to talk about: since she had found out she was going to die, "we have our answer about what's going to happen: it's final."

Curious to learn if she wanted to be able to talk to her parents like she once had, I asked what effect it might have to speak with them about dying. She said she thought it would be devastating for them, and that they're all pretending it's not happening, as it's too painful. I hypothesized that this was about protection—of one another and also oneself. She agreed. So if talking about death is not possible or wanted, are there things she would want to talk to her parents about? Priya told me she has lots of things she feels she needs to say to them before she dies. She wanted to thank them, she wanted to check they were going to be ok, she wanted to laugh with them about silly things, like they used to, she wanted to eat her mother's signature dish. I wrote each one of these down as she spoke, and we set about making a "talking plan". Had Priya had longer, I may have attempted to work towards bringing the family together to be able to speak with one another and potentially allow a joint sharing of sorrow and worry, as they had previously found this helpful. This was not possible, and therefore the focus of our list was what felt possible in that moment and without the luxury of time.

Priya decided the first thing she wanted to do was to start laughing with her parents again, and she chose some YouTube videos she thought they might find funny. I heard from her that being able to laugh and have closeness while watching these videos felt very special. She asked her mother to bring in her curry, which also had the added benefit of reducing how often her mother asked if she was eating. Priya saw how happy it made her to watch her eat homemade food, even if just a little, and we spoke about the memories it conjured for her. Finally, Priya wanted to tackle saying thank you and asking if they were going to be ok. I offered to support her with this, to think about how she might like to start the conversation and how it might be possible. Priya didn't feel in a position to have this conversation verbally, so she decided writing might be the best solution. She spoke about a "goodbye" letter with great sadness, so I reframed this to call it a thank-you letter. We spoke a little about if she had written thank-you letters before, and she decided not to sign it off with goodbye but rather, "love always".

I received the news one morning that Priya's condition had deteriorated, and her death was imminent. Feeling a need to acknowledge our work together and let her know it meant something to me, I wrote her a letter, in the form of a poem (Behan, 2003). Following the work of Behan and the concept of "poetic speech", I used her direct words that I had written down during our sessions to formulate a poem. It didn't take me long to compose something. I went up to her room. She was conscious but very weak. Kindly her parents left the room and gave us a few moments alone, I asked if she had given them the letter, and she nodded. I read her the poem. As with many of these young people I have worked with who have died, endings always seem suboptimal. Perhaps this is something to do with my own sense of loss or denial at these points. For Priya and me, we were quickly interrupted by a nurse; this led to a quick goodbye, and I left the room.

Overall, I had six sessions with Priya over three weeks. I did my best to effect some small shift or change during those last few weeks. Some of my initial hopes at referral for Priya—to be able to have in-depth conversations again with her family, for her family to be able to speak with her and share or offer reassurance—weren't possible. Within the limits and restraints of such a referral, I did my best to slightly open the door to communication at the most impossible time. What we did manage to achieve, I hope, offered Priya some comfort at the end of her life.

Reflections

Working with young adults and their families at times of great distress I have learnt how as "an-other", separate from their existing system, I am in a position to offer a space to pause and reflect on how communication and relationships are working in this new context. What separates us as humans from our animal counterparts is our meta-cognition and ability to step back and reflect on our own thinking and actions. This offers the possibility of effecting change on how life may be working. During periods of stress and trauma our ability to reflect may be impacted; we are consumed by our felt experience, and this can stop us functioning as we may have done previously. Working in oncology, we cannot attempt to remove pain and suffering entirely but offer some small shifts that may support people to feel more resilient in difficult times. What has appeared to be a constant in my talking with people is that when feeling particularly out of control, fearful, or distressed, one looks to another for comfort and strength. When these connections are disrupted, this can be particularly challenging.

When working with those at the end of life, I have found that it is not fear about death per se that appears to be uppermost in people's minds but, rather, the fear of missing family and their family missing them. The privilege of working with someone when they're dying, to be invited into their world, has driven me to want to continue to work hard to support people to reconnect with family, friends, and networks in their lives that give them meaning and a sense of belonging. In order to do this work, however, I have found that I also need to remain connected to others—to a thoughtful and supportive team of like-minded colleagues, to interested and empathetic supervisors, and to the significant people in my life outside work. This work, although hugely rewarding at times, also brings with it the sadness and loss for those young people you have connected with and who have died. I still remain connected to them, without consciously doing so: they remain firmly in my mind and inspire me in what I do.

CHAPTER FIVE

Cancer in adolescence from a trauma perspective

Daniel Glazer

Receiving a diagnosis of cancer can understandably be highly distressing, and many young people experience moments during treatment when they feel their life is in imminent danger. Psychological ideas and therapeutic approaches that focus on trauma can often help when working with these experiences. Ranging from the cognitive neuroscience models of Brewin, Gregory, Lipton, and Burgess (2010) and van der Kolk (2014), to trauma therapies, such as eye movement desensitisation and reprocessing (EMDR), and integrative approaches drawing on compassion and sensory-motor systems (Fisher, 2017), these models can play an important role in making sense of and working with the trauma of cancer.

However, alongside these ideas, cancer can also be experienced as an existential trauma, as it shakes the foundations of safety, certainty, and meaning that ordinarily help life feel manageable and within our grasp. All the more, for adolescents this happens at a time of life when they are discovering and learning more about themselves and their preferred ways of "being-in-the-world" (Heidegger, 1962).

This chapter reflects on the impact of cancer from a trauma perspective, how young people are impacted by facing mortality, and the ways they learn to live alongside the reality that life is precious, vulnerable, and finite. Alongside the traumatic nature of such an experience, this can lead to a form of personal growth, a dedication to live life according to their values, and the discovery of new ways of *being-in-the world*.

DOI: 10.4324/9781003325475-6

The shattering of the "assumptive world"

In order to obtain a diagnosis of post-traumatic stress disorder, a person needs to have been exposed to or witnessed an event whereby one's life or personal integrity has been threatened. Following this, one might experience flashbacks, hyperarousal, avoidance of reminders of the trauma, and a change in their sense of self (Brewin et al., 2010). It is often the case that, upon hearing the word "cancer", thoughts of dying are the first to enter one's mind, and it is not uncommon for people to get flashbacks from the moment of diagnosis or at difficult points throughout their treatment. However, the threat from hearing the word cancer is not one of imminent danger and is something different from the immediate trauma of, for example, being in a car crash and fearing death at the moment of impact. In helping to explain what happens here, Edmund Husserl, the nineteenth-century philosopher and founder of phenomenology, described what he called the "explosion of the *noema*" (Yalom, 2017): *noema* being a Greek word meaning the content of a thought, judgement, or perception. The exploding *noema* is the moment an internal reality cannot reconcile something that is happening externally. For many young people and their families, receiving a cancer diagnosis is a devastating moment that can shatter long-standing and stable assumptions about self and world (Janoff-Bulman, 1992). These assumptions are shaped by experience, culture, and context, and are akin to Bowlby's notion of "internal working models" (Bowlby, 1979; Brennan, 2001). Our assumptive world does not only contain representations of the self and the world, it also retains a way of making sense of death and mortality.

When working with teenagers, I often find my mind connecting with my own experience of adolescence. I recall my first holiday abroad with friends, at the age of 17. Once away and swayed by peer pressure and a youthful sense of adventure and invisibility, I spent the two weeks riding around the treacherous, winding streets on a rented moped, travelling between the beach and our accommodation. Fortunately, my friends and I all left unharmed, but I've since been struck by this sense that I had of a protective shell. I held assumptions that bad things would not happen to me, but should something terrible have happened, my "*noema*" would perhaps have "exploded". Certain assumptions we can hold, particularly in adolescence—such as those of fairness, justice, and that bad things do not happen to good people—can suddenly, in one stroke, be shattered when receiving a cancer diagnosis.

Being faced with a sudden and life-affecting trauma can expose the fragility of life. For instance, Michael, a young father, would highlight to me how one minute he was holding his daughter's hand on the way to school, and the next moment he was holding it on a paediatric cancer ward. It is breath-taking at times to think how quickly life can change. Existential phenomenology proposes that uncertainty is a constant of existence. It expresses itself in those surprising and extraordinary moments, but it is always there lurking in every moment that passes (Spinelli, 2014). Cancer, regardless of prognosis, can shatter the structures of safety and certainty we put around life. This short vignette of a meeting with Mohamed highlights this process:

Mohamed

Mohamed was 18 years old, with a diagnosis of leukaemia; a long and arduous treatment, but his prognosis was good. After nearly three years, he was approaching the final stages of treatment, and everyone was congratulating his pragmatic attitude and determination that had carried him though the process. However, Mohamed found himself struggling with intense anxiety at the point his treatment was finishing. It was following an "anxiety attack" during an appointment with his consultant that he sought a referral to the Psych-Oncology Team. During our first session he exclaimed, "I took everything cancer threw at me and beat it, but now, when I'm able to get back to life, I'm suffering with horrible anxiety. I don't get it."

I spent this initial session getting to know Mohamed and learnt that he had always loved football and he had been the captain of his school team before his cancer diagnosis. In helping to explain his experience of anxiety, he told me it was like stepping up to take a penalty kick in a big match:

"Usually I would put the ball on the spot, take a few steps back, and pick my spot. I take a deep breath, focus, and then take the shot. Finishing treatment feels like taking a penalty, but this time it's like my legs going wobbly, I can't decide where to hit the ball, and I end up missing the goal completely."

"So usually you would be cool and calm under pressure, but now it feels like the moment is getting the better of you?" I replied, trying to imagine what that must feel like.

"Yes, something like that", Mohamed responded.

"So something about this moment of coming to the end of treatment feels like missing a penalty?" I asked.

Mohamed sat back, and I could see him examining the connection in his mind. "No, not missing a penalty, it's more the feeling of being so terrified that I can't even take the penalty."

Holding on to my curiosity, I enquired further: "What is it about the penalty kick specifically that feels so terrifying? Is it a fear of missing, what other people might think if you do, or something else completely?"

Mohamed's eyes lit up, and he saw a connection almost straight away: "Well, now that I think of it, a penalty kick can feel like the most important thing in the world: when you step up, it's like life or death, the only thing in the world that matters at that moment."

I was struck by how Mohamed appeared to be struggling with issues of "life or death" at the end of treatment. Naively perhaps, my assumption was that this struggle would more likely occur at the beginning of treatment. Mohamed went on to tell me that he had just been so focused on "getting through it", it had not really hit him that on a number of occasions he was close to dying. What we went on to consider together was that Mohamed was once again in that "*noema*"-shattering moment, questioning how to live, when all the structures he had put around life and assumptions he held were no longer as valid as they once were. Just like a penalty kick, Mohamed had lived by the notion, "If I stay strong and focused, I can score and win." This may be a great philosophy for life, and certainly one that had helped Mohamed score penalties and in many ways cope with his arduous treatment. However, Mohamed had now arrived at a place where this no longer made sense to him entirely. The question for our work was how Mohamed could hold on to values of achievement and "winning"—values that were important to him—while also incorporating his new understanding of the inherent uncertainties of life.

Working with people whose assumptive world ("*noema*") has been shattered is, in my view, something that, as professionals, we struggle greatly to get to grips with. One challenge is that it causes us to come face to face with our own mortality, and despite the stories we tell ourselves, that we, too, are vulnerable to the uncertainties of living. Here are some ideas that might help in considering how to prepare, be with or reflect on connections with young people gripped by existential trauma:

» What existential tensions might arise in you, the professional, meeting this young person? This might be a sense of meaninglessness, vulnerability, uncertainty, isolation, or, more generally, death anxiety.

» How does this present in your body? We will experience these tensions in our body in all sorts of ways, from a deep churning in the gut to a desire to want to avoid, look away, or flee.

» How can you stay present rather than pulled away by these forces? If you completely avoid and cut off from these tensions, then it will be harder to be present with someone and offer something therapeutic in relation to their experience.

» How can you soothe your body in these moments?

» Remembering to stay curious. The other person's experience, knowledge assumptions, perspective, and history are different from your own. Anxiety and fear will mean that your curiosity, creativity, and energy is dampened, leading you to turn towards more certain and prescriptive ways of being, which may not fit with someone you are offering support to.

» Stay connected to notions of a shared humanity—that we are all "fellow travellers" in dealing with issues of existence (Yalom, 2002).

The centrality of meaning to trauma

Having completed training in EMDR, a trauma-focused therapy, I volunteered to pick up referrals where the request for psychology input was to support a young person with "nightmares", "flashbacks", or other experiences of unwanted reliving of cancer treatment. A fundamental part of this approach, along with other models such as existential phenomenology, is a focus on meaning being central to experience.

A great deal has been written on the neurobiology of trauma (for a review, see Brewin et al., 2010). The focus of this understanding is that the heighted sense of arousal during a life-threatening experience dampens the hippocampus, which is responsible for encoding context and time and creating a verbal narrative, while the amygdala, which encodes the sensory and emotional experiences, is activated. This creates a fractured memory whereby the sensory and emotional aspects of an experience can be activated in the absence of narrative and context that help make sense of it. Although this process helps one to understand flashbacks and is a guide towards interventions, it seems that there is an additional phenomenological step to be considered. What is someone's experience of cancer? What does it mean to them, and how are they making sense of certain moments that are experienced as traumatic?

In helping to make sense of this, I share the story of Jonny, who was diagnosed with cancer at the age of 17.

Jonny

I first met Jonny during his treatment for leukaemia, and our contact ended when he recovered and no longer needed to visit the hospital so regularly.

A few years later, I received an email from Jonny, asking if he could come and see me again, as he was having some trouble dealing with life at university. When I saw Jonny in the waiting room, I barely recognized him. I hadn't seen him since his treatment and recalled a thin, sickly boy who was fed up and missed his ordinary life. In front of me now was a healthy, tall, strong young man. He leapt up off the seat and we greeted each other warmly, both revelling for a moment at the time that had passed.

Once sat down, I asked Jonny to catch me up on the last few years. Despite having cancer during his A-Levels, Jonny had managed to pass with straight A's and was now in his first year studying law at a top university. He beamed with pride at being the first person to go to university in his family. Jonny told me that he had a boyfriend, and that they had been together for six months. We had spoken about sexuality before and recalled him being deeply concerned that he might die, never having kissed another boy. "I've kissed a girl, but that doesn't count any more", I remembered him telling me. I was moved by where he had got to in life compared to where he had been when I last saw him.

"So, how come you got in touch again, Jonny, how can I be of help?" I asked.

Jonny told me that despite the progress he had made, he was struggling with daily flashbacks and nightmares connected to his time following a bone marrow transplant. His nightmares centred on being in prison, and at every turn there were gangs of men who wanted to kill him. They would hurl abuse at him, call him names, and tell him all the things they were going to do. Jonny would wake up regularly in the middle of the night in a sweat, heart racing, fearing for his life.

We talked more about the time on treatment and which moments were coming to him as flashbacks. Jonny described a time after his transplant, when he was so weak and sick he thought he couldn't go on any more.

The formulation we worked on together was that if we processed this time during treatment, this would mean that his body would not feel as stuck with this sense of imminent danger, and his flashbacks and nightmares would heal. After a few sessions of EMDR treatment, his sense of safety did improve: cognitively, he could tell himself he was now safe, but he was still in a heighted physiological state when thinking about that time. There was something else keeping his anxiety stuck.

In EMDR there is a technique called the "float-back" or "somatic bridge", whereby you invite someone to connect with an emotional or bodily sensation and see if anything resonates from an earlier experience. We connected in to the feeling in his body when he thought about the time he had felt so physically weak on the ward.

I knew Jonny had been brought up by his dad, a single parent for a while, before he remarried. Jonny started to tell me how the feeling in his body is the same as when he recalled being 7 years old, and his mother packed her bags to leave the family home. He recalled his mum shoving him to the floor as he tried to cling on to stop her stuffing clothes into the suitcase. His pleas, however, were futile, and she left him alone for seven hours before his dad came home from work. "Those seven hours alone felt as long as the six weeks in recovery from my transplant", he told me.

With further exploring and processing using an EMDR framework, to my surprise, the main issue connecting his nightmares, flashbacks, and previous experiences was not fear and a sense of death being around the corner: it was shame. The 7-year-old part of Jonny carried the story of feeling weak and vulnerable. When faced with moments of physical weakness and isolation after his bone marrow transplant, the felt sense of the experience resonated, and the 7-year-old part of Jonny saw this new experience in the same way.

Jonny, now a wise young man, was able to reflect on how he had always pushed this part of himself away—seeing it as "pathetic"—unwittingly further isolating and rejecting a part of him that was looking for connection and safety.

The nightmares and flashbacks stopped relatively quickly after Jonny was able to identify what 7-year-old Jonny needed, and how his now young adult self could accept and offer compassion to this part of him to soothe his feelings of shame. For Jonny, the earlier experience of his mother leaving was intricately connected in the meaning and resonance of being on the ward. These moments on the ward were held almost in stasis, encoded as painful emotional and bodily memories that were being regularly re-experienced in the form of nightmares and flashbacks. Therefore, the idiosyncratic meaning of an experience is paramount in shaping an experience as traumatic.

A broader perspective on meaning

Reflecting on how Jonny was making sense of his experiences was a vital part of the therapeutic process. One role of the therapist is to help someone "begin to consider, from the standpoint of their own lived experience, what their meanings provide with regard to the 'life-stories' constructed for themselves" (Spinelli, 1997, p. 16). However, when working with issues of mortality, even meaning can sometimes feel somewhat limited. Do we grasp on to meaning—any meaning—to provide a sliver of comfort and security when we are "standing naked in the storm of life" (Becker, 1973, p. 86)? In this connection, Spinelli (2014) considers the role of meaninglessness when working with meaning (i.e., the meaninglessness of our meanings). This can result in landing at a place where meanings perhaps do not need to be held so tightly, with so much certainty and conviction.

Therefore, although identifying meaning is central to therapeutic work in this area, it also seems important to consider how meanings are being held and the strength of the connection to them. As such, another role of the therapist can be to support meanings being held in a way that respects their transience, developing a more flexible connection to them. So, Jonny held tightly on to a belief of the importance of being strong. If this were to shift and he were to develop a new belief in relation to his experiences, it would perhaps be important to hold this new belief, not with the same firm grip, but with an understanding that meanings change and fade with context and time.

Reflecting on how meaning may be held in ways other than language and narrative is another consideration when taking a broader perspective on meaning. Trauma has been described as an "experience beyond words" (Meichenbaum, 2012). Neurobiologically, our emotional and sensory systems are heightened, while our thinking brain is taken offline. This means that language-based narrative and meaning can be limited when making sense of trauma. Bessel van der Kolk (2014) famously described how "the body keeps the score", meaning that the body holds on to the memories in physiological states. Indeed, when asked about a cancer experience, many young people describe physiological responses, such as a feeling of dread in their gut. This can be experienced as a deep, churning feeling, and it is not uncommon to see young people with their arms wrapped about their stomach, hunched over, when talking or thinking about their treatment. Of course, other bodily reactions can also occur, such as a racing heart, sweaty palms, or parasympathetic reactions, such as fatigue, feeling spaced out, or numbness. During trauma therapy, it is often seen that these reactions, such as "dread in the gut", connect to moments during treatment when someone is in a particularly perilous state and is fearing the worst. Therefore, meaning is central to trauma, but it is important to broaden our perspective on meaning and to pay particular attention to embodied responses as well as verbally accessible narratives.

A new way of "being-in-the-world"

Following trauma such as a cancer experience, when assumptions about the self and world have been challenged, integration of new knowledge and experience needs to be woven into a coherent narrative of the self and the world. In other words, if we always thought that life was fair and under our control, how do we move forward with an awareness that life is inherently unpredictable?

Adolescence is a turbulent and exciting time of risk-taking, trying out new experiences, and experimenting with new versions of the self. Perhaps one of the great misunderstandings of the self, who we are, our identity, is the idea that we reach completion once we are fully-fledged "grown-ups". Adolescence is really just the start. Polkinghorne (1988) describes how the self is experienced not as a static entity, but as a process of *becoming*. Similarly, White and Epston (1990) argue that each person becomes his or her story, with identity defined through that narrative.

Therefore, it is a hopeful reminder that the self is always in the process of *becoming*, and one task of the therapist following a trauma is to facilitate the integration of new knowledge into an updated storyline of the self and the world. The therapist achieves this goal through a transformational dialogue that acts to destabilize, deconstruct, and defamiliarize the clients' consciously presented narrative of self (McLeod, 1997). I highlight this process through my work with Amber:

Amber

I first met Amber about a year after her treatment for a brain tumour at the age of 17. She walked into the therapy room using a crutch, sat down, and signed deeply. She told me how tired she was: even the walk from the waiting area made her out of breath and exhausted. If it wasn't the fatigue stopping her doing things, it was the recovery from a left-sided paralysis. She told me how hard she tried to keep up with her friends, joining them on nights out and shopping. Amber relayed to me a recent story of a night out with friends. She wore her favourite outfit, and for a moment felt like the old Amber. She had picked up her crutch, stared at her reflection in the mirror, and started to cry. The crutch was aptly named, she thought to herself: it told everyone she was helpless and weak. She threw it onto her bed and left home without it, limping out the door. Her friends were kind, giving her the seat on the train and letting her lean on them as they walked to the club. But each kind gesture confirmed Amber's sense of herself as weak, and she silently raged inside. After about 30 minutes in the club, the music was piercing her mind, the alcohol she consumed against medical advice was starting to take hold, and her exhaustion started to feel like a thousand kilos on her shoulders. "I blacked-out", she told me. Amber did not remember anything that happened next, but a friend told her she fainted and, luckily, was physically caught so she did not crash to the floor. We spoke about that night some more, and Amber told me that she remembered lying in the ambulance and hating herself for not being able to "just cope". After being given the all clear by the doctors in A&E at 5 a.m., Amber made her way home with her mother, who was furious that she had gone out without her crutch.

After a few sessions, Amber started to tell me more about her life. She had been devastated at a young age, when her father left. He would often drink and was verbally abusive, but to young Amber he was her dad, and she desperately wanted his love and affection. After he left, contact was sporadic for the rest of her young life. He would occasionally call on birthdays or, if not, he would send a card. Sometimes she would hear her mother shouting down the phone at him to be more present for his daughter. Amber tucked away her hurt and became brilliant at virtually everything she did. She was bright, sporty, popular, creative, musical, and theatrical. However, Amber never felt good about her achievements—to her they weren't even achievements at all. She would chase the praise, but it never filled the hole. She needed to become better and better, it was unrelenting and it never worked. Her sense of personal devastation at not being able to be on this night out like old Amber started to make sense.

After a few months after our first meeting, Amber found out that she had not been selected for an important position at school. She was devastated and angry, and despite my attempts to think about what this meant to her, I could not reach her. She was furious at the teachers for not seeing the effort she was putting in, and no one understood how she felt—not her mum, her partner, her friends, and certainly not me!

Amber, through her narrative, was describing to me that cancer had meant that she now saw herself weak, and, to her, being weak meant that she would not be loved and she would be ultimately rejected. This meaning can be derived from her descriptions of the night out, her dad leaving, and, finally, not being given this important position at school. As such, "The remembered past reflects the current views we hold about ourselves" (Spinelli, 1997, p. 45). However, the narrative also gives clues to a preferred way of *being* or a direction she wished to move towards. Upon closer discussion, Amber highlighted that she wanted to be accepted despite perceived imperfections, to feel *good-enough* even though she occupied a body that challenged her notion of this.

Using her description of *Old Amber* provided a window to explore this further. We considered what aspects of *Old Amber* she wanted to hold on to, and what she wanted to let go of. Importantly, Amber highlighted that, rather than being *New Amber*, she wanted to think of herself as *Still Amber*.

This declaration beautifully encapsulated that she was "Still" the same Amber, with the same values and passion for living fully, while also, at times, wanting to be "Still" and slow down.

> A few months later Amber's dad called her mobile phone. Ordinarily, if she spoke to him, she would be polite, eager to please, and accepting of any unkind words she received down the phone—*Old Amber*. This time was different though. Amber's experience of being-in-the-world (Heidegger, 1962) was starting to shift. As such, she was bravely venturing out with her crutch or saying no to social engagements when she didn't feel up to it. When her dad called that day, she was tired and was experiencing pain down her left leg. The last thing she needed was to absorb her dad's mindless grievances. She interrupted him talking about how she never called or visited: "I'm not little Amber any more, dad, you can't just call me up and have a go at me and expect me to come running." Amber politely told him that she was tired and would call him back another time. Upon putting the phone down, Amber rested well on the sofa, feeling a weight lift off her. Perhaps slightly overtaken by the moment, I was considering why she hadn't gone further, and I was silently wishing she had unleashed all her rage, telling him exactly what she felt. Perhaps, seeing my expression, Amber, in a short but thoughtful statement, reminded me that our job is to travel with a client to a destination of their choosing, rather than taking them where we feel they should go. "I know some people would say I should tell him exactly what I think, but that's just not me, I am *Still Amber*, after all", she told me with a grin.

In considering how to move forward from a cancer experience, it is tempting to think about how to fix it and go back to how things had been. Indeed, when working with young people, we might often hear, "I just want to be that carefree 12-year-old again". However, the process of integrating experiences into a new and updated way of being is perhaps akin to the Japanese art of *Kintsugi,* which involves repairing broken pottery. This is both a craft and a philosophy about breakage being part of the history of an object and not something that should be disguised. In Kintsugi there is an embracing of the imperfect, and repairs are illuminated rather than hidden. Consequently, through this process of integration, young people like Amber have taught me that they will often do the work and piece together old narratives and values with new and preferred ways of being, connecting their experiences with new ideas and possibilities. Indeed, Amber continued to use her crutch but went on to embrace it as symbol of comfort, security, and resolve, rather than a sign of weakness.

The process of integrating experiences into a preferred narrative of self is not one that comes without difficulty or hazards. Just like any journey, the road can at times be bumpy or even treacherous. It is not easy to integrate a traumatic cancer experience into a new way of being. For some, this might move them into a more nihilistic place—"what's the point if we are all going to die anyway"—which might result in a chronic lack of motivation and low mood. The flip side might be a more existential rebellion—"I could have died, so I now need to live life fully all the time"—which, although can be enriching, can also be stressful and exhausting.

I was recently working with a young man of 23 who had been through a series of medical issues, one after the other, since he was 15 years old. Following these experiences, he was determined that this was not going to hold him back, and surviving meant that he would "live life to the max". I had always greatly admired the way he said yes to every opportunity and his life had become filled with interesting people and experiences. However, when COVID struck, he came to realize that although this was a great strength, the conviction with which he held his new "live life to the max" belief was perhaps undermining his ability to cope with lockdown, even after everything he had been through. Therefore, when incorporating experiences and meanings into a new and updated way of being-in-the-world (Heidegger, 1962), it seems important to be able to hold a light touch and curiosity towards these new beliefs. After all, change is always happening.

A note on posttraumatic growth

As young people finish treatment, they move into end of treatment clinics and, all being well, into what are often called "Late Effects" Services (see chapter 6). Although cancer is often thought about as an acute condition, its effects can, in fact, be chronic. From cognitive changes to chronic fatigue, fertility issues to managing amputations, the physical changes can be devastating and can require lasting management. However, although there can be psychological difficulties during this period, what is seen time and again is a form of psychological maturity. Often in the literature this is referred to as posttraumatic growth (Kilmer, 2006).

Posttraumatic growth is a construct that aims to encapsulate the experience of those who endure trauma and yet still experience positive growth, which is transformative and goes beyond coping (Kilmer, 2006). Posttraumatic growth aims not to ignore or discount the potentially negative and highly distressing effects of traumatic experiences but, rather, to capture individual experience that features growth and change out of adversity.

There have been countless examples of this form of post-traumatic growth in my work with young people.

Jamie, a gifted musician, struggled with anxiety during and after treatment for a brain tumour. However, despite being cognitively and physically slowed down, he described how he now played his guitar with more rhythm and feeling. He had not only integrated his physical changes alongside a preferred identity, his experience had helped him to grow into a different—and, he would argue, improved—musician.

Similarly, Amber (described above) let me know that she did not "sweat over the small stuff" any more, such as how she looked or whether people like her: she felt more comfortable and able to present her true self to the world.

Ismail, a 22-year-old young man who had Hodgkin's lymphoma as a teenager, saw a number of his friends die of their cancers. "I owe it to them to live my life to the full", he told me. He subsequently faced some of his fears, including asking out a new partner, leaving his job that was meant to be just a stop-gap, and following his dreams into a new career. He also jumped out of a plane!

It seems that an experience of having to face and grapple with mortality at a young age can have deep and meaningful effects. Indeed, an evaluation at University College London Hospital demonstrated that young adults treated for cancer as teenagers experienced positive social, emotional, and quality-of life-adjustment. This connects with Irvin Yalom's famous maxim: "Though the physicality of death destroys us the idea of death can save us" (Yalom, 2002, p. 7). When faced with an awareness of existential issues, in particular an awareness of our own mortality, this can lead to profound psychological growth.

One role of the professional is to listen to the multiple stories that young people are telling and ensure we are paying attention to the full experience. Alongside cancer being an experience of loss and suffering, it is important also to hear those other stories, the ones that are mentioned more rarely but involve growth and "metamorphosis" (Fredman & Dalal, 1998).

Final words

My hope here has been to convey a set of ideas and principles that connects to my work and young people's experiences of cancer. Through my work, I try as best as I can to hold a therapeutic stance of "curiosity" (Cecchin, 1987) or what is called "unknowing" (Spinelli, 1997) in existential phenomenology—in other words, attempting to understand the world of another, as far as that is possible, while recognizing that my worldview and experience are different from theirs.

Therefore, my intention has not been to convey a "truth" that young people always go through certain processes, or that it is always possible to uncover these through exploration. It has not been my intention to imply that these processes occur in a predetermined, linear fashion—for example, from a traumatic shattering of the assumptive world to integrating these experiences into a new way of being. Finally, it is also not my intention to be communicating that growth and positive change will always happen or, if they do, happen neatly. Rather, my hope has been to communicate ideas that help ground me in this work and provide a framework for exploring, understanding, and healing.

It is impossible to separate ourselves from therapeutic work that resonates profoundly. It can be hard to acknowledge the reality that these are young people faced with such uncertainty about their lives. They come face to face with an awareness of death at such a young age and respond to this in a multitude of ways. We, the professionals in this field, are then only one step removed from this (and you the reader now two steps). Although we are not experiencing what the young person in front of us is going though, I find it helpful to hold on to the idea that we are "fellow travellers" (Yalom, 2002) in grappling with issues of existence, suffering, and purpose. This can help to create a therapeutic relationship that strives towards something akin to what Martin Buber calls the I-Thou relationship (Cooper, 2017). This is one in which there is a meeting of people who are connected by their shared humanity: a relationship in which healing from trauma can occur.

CHAPTER SIX

Reverberations through the mind: explorations of emotional complexities arising from childhood cancer and its "late effects"

Petra A. M. Mohr

W hat does it mean to be diagnosed with cancer as a child—a disease that, in the collective mind as well as often in the individual's reality, is associated with death? Even if the prognosis is good, the child's mind is likely to be faced with death on some level: through an inner sense of how ill her body is, through sensing it in the minds of loved others who fear for her, or through seeing other ill children on the ward. How does it affect your sense of others when you are being treated by doctors and nurses who want to help you and cure you, yet the treatment they give you often feels intrusive and damaging to your inner bodily core? What does it mean to be given treatment that involves toxic chemicals being pumped into your body, being beamed with invisible but dangerous rays, having parts of your body taken out or limbs removed, being given someone else's bone marrow—all in an attempt to save your life?

In this chapter I explore themes of how cancer and cancer treatment can affect a child emotionally and leave traces in the deep layers of the mind, traces that can re-awaken at later periods of stress and upheaval.

I explore these issues through discussing psychotherapeutic work with young people referred by the Late Effects Clinic to our Psych-Oncology Team. The Late Effects Clinic works with people who have had cancer when younger and have been in remission for longer than five years. "Late effects" refers to effects that can develop after having cancer treatment such as chemotherapy and radiotherapy and can include reduced growth,

DOI: 10.4324/9781003325475-7

increased risk of heart problems and infertility, and impact on cognitive functioning.

Specifically, I speak about young people who had some form of cancer when they were babies or children and who are now between 18 and 24 and hence, by age, on the cusp of adulthood, but who find themselves unable to move forward into what normally constitutes leading an adult life. The transition to adulthood seems to be a particular trigger point in which elements from the deeper layers of the mind may rise up into consciousness and impact on the development of identity, on emotions and outlook on life (and death), on attitudes towards being helped, and sometimes leading to darker states of mind.

I have collated some of the main themes that have arisen in my clinical work with such young people and have developed composite vignettes that illustrate these themes. I use composite vignettes from work with parents of children going through treatment for cancer and who have been supported by the Psych-Oncology Team. Childhood cancer has a traumatizing impact on the whole family, creating massive emotional pressures and paradoxes that can reverberate through their lives for years to come. Specifically, I explore four themes: guilt, the search for causes, a discontinuity in biographical narrative, and paradoxes. In addition, by looking at the potential impact of cancer and its treatment on a very young mind, I outline the specific difficulties for young people whose cancer treatment happened during infancy.

A trauma in early childhood might impact on the person's future life in hidden ways. They might automatically react to certain sensual experiences (such as particular smells) or situational ones (such as seeing a doctor) with panic, without understanding why. If they underwent cancer treatment as very young children, there might be thoughts and fantasies and associations that were formed during the pre-verbal period. These—"sense-less" without the help of language and the understanding of another person— continue to lie unprocessed in the unconscious, potentially influencing future emotional responses.

Looking for causes

It is in our human nature to strive for meaning and explanations for random events. We feel unsettled if we do not know why something has happened, and being overcome with grave events outside our control can be terrifying. We look for reasons, even if this involves finding a reason to blame ourselves. If it is my fault, at least there is a hope that I can change it. With many of the young people I have met through the

Psych-Oncology work who have or have had cancer, the question of "why me?" lurks somewhere in their mind.

Chloe

Chloe, a young adult, had leukaemia as a child. She has recently met a young man whom she likes, but she is scared of starting a relationship. She is scared of being intimate. She does not feel comfortable in her body and thinks her body is ugly. She would love to have a family one day, but she does not know whether the chemotherapy she had as a child has destroyed her fertility. Even if she could conceive, she is frightened. She feels her body is "damaged goods"—damaged through cancer and its treatment. In her fantasy, her womb is toxic and is no place for a growing foetus, and even if a baby would survive, she believes that her child would be killed later by cancer, because she would have passed down her "bad genes".

When she was a child, nobody had explained to Chloe what exactly was going on. She knows that her parents and the doctors wanted to protect her from the truth, but that left her with her own ideas and fantasies. She must have been a bad child to be given such a bad illness. Now, as an adult, she is still ruminating over this question: "Why did I get cancer? Was it something I did? Was I punished for being bad? Was I born bad?"

Such "irrational" explanations and fantasies that individuals might have are also represented on a collective level. Perceiving cancer as punishment is not uncommon and often lingers inside the person's mind just outside their awareness (Carbone, 1996). Vrinten and colleagues (2017), conducting a meta-analysis of 102 studies from various countries about people's fears about cancer, found that, where religion is felt as being important, there are common ideas of cancer being part of God's plan or test. Vrinten and colleagues found that:

Participants talked about cancer as if it were not just a disease, but a sentient persona with malicious personality traits, such as viciousness, unpredictability, and indestructibility . . . [as something that is] lurking inside you, spreading stealthily and inescapably. [Vrinten et al., 2017, p. 1073]

They describe how there seems to be an association with betrayal. These ideas arise due to the fact that in the early stages of most cancers there are no accompanying physical symptoms. The cancer stays hidden, and then, once revealed, it is too late. Further common ideas are of cancer as a parasite, and the images of cancerous growth as burning, rotting, or being eaten away from the inside. Other perceptions that abound, for example within traditional healer cultures, are of cancer being caused by bad blood or bad air. In the United Kingdom and other countries some people believe (against rational knowledge) that cancer is contagious, or that it is caused by moral wrong-doing such as adultery, or by trauma such as divorce (Dein, 2004). The UK media and some charity campaigns often use war metaphors when speaking about cancer. The idea that cancer is an enemy can lead to the person thinking that they have to be strong and fight all the time, with the implication that if they feel weak, or if they might not survive, they have not been fighting hard enough. Cancer treatment is then imagined as an army fighting the aggressive enemy inside one's body (Judd, 2013). Several of the young adults I have worked with who have had cancer when they were little have spoken about how they feel as if there is something wrong and anti-life inside them, and they cannot make any tangible connection to explain why they are feeling that way:

Kieron

Kieron can't stand all this talk about "fighting cancer" and being a "survivor of cancer". As a teenager, he had not told any of his peers that he had had cancer. He hated others feeling sorry for him. Looking back, he hates himself for having put up with all the intrusive treatment. He thinks his younger self should have been stronger and feels ashamed for having been so powerless. Kieron hates it when people say to him "well done" for having fought off the cancer. "They say I survived, but I haven't. I died." He feels very much as if he is just existing now. He often feels depressed and lethargic "without reason". When in such a state of mind, he isolates himself and has no contact with others or the outside world. His mind then seems to "disappear" into a lifeless place, where he doesn't care about anyone or anything, a state of mind where the passing of time, thoughts, even his physical needs don't matter any more.

Trying to find a reason that their child contracted cancer is also something many of the parents we work with talk to us about.

Mr and Ms Oyekan

Mr and Ms Oyekan are tormented by questions of "why?". Was it their genes, their family line, that passed on the cancer to their child? Has Ms Oyekan passed it on in her breast milk? Have they used mobile phones too much around their child? Given their child the wrong food? Or have they done something to offend God that caused this punishment?

In the midst of this arbitrary event of a child getting cancer, being faced with the utter sense of powerlessness, trying to find reasons, and blaming themselves might be a way to feel they have some control in an uncontrollable situation. Blaming oneself constitutes an attempt to hold on to something to make sense in the senselessness, and to rail against the fact that, fundamentally, this *should not* happen, this really *is not* right.

Guilt

Trying to find an explanation and blaming oneself can lead to guilt: guilt for somehow being responsible for the cancer, as if one had caused it. A common theme among my conversations with young people with late effects has been a sense of guilt towards their parents for "putting them through" all the worries:

Chloe

Chloe's parents had separated around the time when Chloe had her treatment. In her fantasy Chloe feels it is her fault that they split up. She also feels guilty for having done things that any ordinary adolescent does, like as eating unhealthy food and drinking alcohol—"as if I hadn't already caused enough worry when I was sick".

When a child goes through cancer treatment, there are many stressors impacting on the family: attending appointments, having to stay with one child in hospital while the other parent stays with the other child at home, financial issues due to having to cut down work, to name but a few. This can trigger guilt in parents.

Mr Arden

Mr Arden feels guilty for having drifted apart from his wife, with both struggling to cope with the stress of their child's long treatment for leukaemia. He feels guilty towards their older child, for not paying the same amount of attention to her. He believes he should have been able to cope better with the whole situation and be a "better" parent and husband.

Guilt towards a sibling for having taken up all the attention is also a common feeling among young people who have had childhood cancer; and siblings, in turn, might feel guilty for being healthy and for having had bad thoughts towards their sick brother or sister. Guilt can permeate the whole family.

There are many losses associated with your child having cancer. There is the loss of the healthy child in the present, as well as a potential loss of a future that might have been, particularly if the child is young and their development is affected. There is the likelihood of the loss of future fertility and hence, for a parent, the potential loss of future grandchildren. Furthermore, there may be losses arising from living with physical disabilities and chronic health conditions. The grief that these losses evoke might in themselves evoke feelings of guilt:

Baby Tamsin

Baby Tamsin received months of intensive treatment, including surgery and radiotherapy. The latest scan showed that the cancer had reduced. The extended family and friends are elated: "Isn't she doing well? What good news!" However, Tamsin's mother cannot feel positive. These latest results will not take away the constant fear of her baby's death, a fear she has been living with since the diagnosis. Not feeling pleased about the good scan results makes her feel guilty. She also feels guilty for grieving for the healthy child that was, and for feeling angry at being robbed of a future of ordinary mother–child interaction. She feels guilty for wishing that she had a different child, a healthy child. Sometimes she even feels angry towards her child, which she knows is irrational, for "making her" constantly be faced with the fear of her child dying. This, then, becomes another source of guilt, for feeling that way.

Feeling guilty for having certain feelings brings me to a form of guilt that can be particularly tenacious and counter to rational knowledge: feeling guilty for having survived.

Keith

Keith, a young adult who had gone through cancer treatment as a baby, has no conscious memory of the treatment, yet whenever he hears of someone's relative having cancer, he feels guilty. Why did he survive and others didn't? He wishes he could swap places. Logically, he knows it is not his fault that his parents went through such great distress, having to live with the fear that he might die. Yet he has been feeling guilty all his life. He cannot tell his parents about this guilt. His parents had fought for his survival—how can he let them know that he sometimes wishes he had died?

With this form of guilt, there can be an accompanying sense of betrayal, the feeling that the person has betrayed the others who did not make it— as if one's survival happens at the expense of someone else's death. The person might have felt relieved for surviving and then felt bad about the relief, knowing that others did not survive. Such conflictual feelings bring a confusing complexity to one's emotional lives:

Anna

Anna had lived on hospital wards for long periods of her childhood. She has memories of other children there. There was a boy she played with. One day there was all this rushing around, and then her friend just disappeared. Anna was left with the confusion of what was going on and up to this day wonders what happened to the boy. Now she understands that he probably died. Why did she survive and he died?

Since leaving school, Anna feels she has not done anything with her life. She feels guilty for wasting her life, for all the worry she has caused her parents as a child with cancer, all the worries she is causing her parents now still. She feels guilty for worrying her parents, guilty for letting down all those who helped her survive, by her now "not being better and getting on with her life", and guilty for not feeling happy. She feels she doesn't deserve to have survived. She feels guilty for not feeling more grateful that she survived when others didn't. She knows that she nearly died and was brought back from the edge. She believes her survival to be a flaw in the universe: as she said to me, "I shouldn't even be here."

Anna does not want to talk to her parents about the traumatic time. She worries about upsetting her parents. She wants to protect them from feeling guilty for not having brought her to the hospital immediately back then. So they do not talk about it, each protecting each other, each carrying their guilt on their own.

Not having acted quickly enough or not having "seen it" is a common feeling among the parents we work with.

Ms Rodriguez

Ms Rodriguez, whose child is going through treatment, constantly thinks back to the time before the diagnosis, when her 8-year-old son complained of leg pain, which she assumed to be muscular strain from playing sports. Ms Rodriguez constantly plays the question in her mind: "What if I had realized sooner that something serious was wrong with my child? Maybe the prognosis would have been better now."

As a parent, one of the hardest things about having a child with cancer is being faced with the inability to protect that child. Having provided nurture, security, and protection from harm to their developing child, they

suddenly are unable to do so. As a mother of a teenager going through cancer treatment once told me: "Before she had the cancer, I used to be able to
kiss everything better." Not being able to make one's child better puts one
in touch with utter helplessness: both parent and child find themselves in
grip of a traumatic situation that happens completely outside their control.

The child's trust and faith in a benign world and their unquestioned
assumption of their parents' protective presence is being shattered. Emanuel, Colloms, Mendelsohn, Muller, and Testa (1990), describing their
psychotherapy work with hospitalized children with leukaemia, state
how young children in particular "expressed profound disillusion in the
previously idealized capacity of their parents to protect them from illness
and intrusion" (p. 30). As explored above, self-blame and guilt might be
a way to offer some illusion of control and might feel preferable to being
emotionally in touch with their powerlessness in this situation.

Trauma in infancy and early childhood

Before I continue with the themes arising in psychotherapy work with
young people who have had childhood cancer, I should like to make a
diversion into what it might mean for an infant to have to undergo cancer
treatment. I do so in order to put into context the narratives of young people who had been treated for cancer when they were infants.

People sometimes believe that an infant will not be very much affected
by a distressing experience because they are too young to remember—as
if the fact of not having conscious memories were a protection against the
impact of the experience. Yet we all know that not understanding what is
happening makes a distressing experience more distressing. In fact, an
infant will not have had the experiences of processing even the ordinary
ups and downs of life. I would like to quote at length from Blomberg
(2005) speaking about premature children:

> Physical experiences (representations) of the struggle for survival
> may remain throughout their lives. They have been subjected to life-
> giving treatment, but this unfortunately includes essential violations
> and examinations that hurt such a little body and that the brain does not
> have a chance to register, systematize, and find out *where* it hurts and
> *where* the danger is coming from. [. . .] Even if parents have been there
> it is still the child itself that has to endure the physical pain. The envi-
> ronment has, in this way, not been able to be facilitating, but rather the
> opposite, i.e. perceived as terrifying by the child. Many children with
> early physical experiences of pain have, despite "good enough mother-
> ing", a deeply-rooted experience in the internal world that mothers and
> fathers are not to be trusted, as they have not been able to protect them

from the unending pain and terror [. . .] The terror is so all-embracing that it cannot be localized in the surrounding world where it can assume the form of an external enemy. The threat is omnipresent, both within and outside the child. [Blomberg, 2005, p. 28; italics as in original]

This account illustrates very well the impact that invasive medical treatment can have on a baby. Freud (1920g, 1926d) describes helplessness as an important feature that makes an experience traumatic. He describes trauma as something that "pierces" our protective shield. In the case of a young child undergoing cancer treatment, they are helpless in dealing with internal perceptions and sensations, as well as those impacting them from the environment. Undergoing cancer treatment, the infant has to manage feeling unwell physically, of pain coming from inside the body and from the medical treatment, side effects such as nausea and altered taste and smell, and changes such as loss of hair, the impact of steroids, or surgery. This is in itself overwhelming—not understanding what is going on makes it so much more difficult and frightening. To a preschool child, taking words literally, "[a] respirator may sound like a monster. [They] may believe surgery is where the doctor will cut them up like vegetables in a salad" (Yehuda, 2016, p. 34). Gaps in comprehension or knowledge of what is happening may be filled with fantasies that can be even more terrifying than reality. In addition to their internal sense of disorder and chaos, the person is faced with an external environment that feels unsafe (Lee & Elfer, 2013). The child's usual security structures are out of sync: their routines and environment have changed, strangers come and go and do things to them, and, most importantly, their parents or carers are different from their usual selves, as they themselves are likely to be frightened, worried, and stressed (which the infant or child will pick up on even when not openly expressed). Witnessing the person you depend on being overwhelmed must be very frightening.

Here it is helpful to consider the psychoanalytic theory of containment originating in Bion's ideas (1959, 1962a, 1962b) and its impact on emotional development. When an infant is overwhelmed with distress, they communicate this via an emotional pathway and "project" the distress onto their caregiver. When open to this emotional communication, the caretakers feel this distress in themselves, try to process this by thinking about "what could the matter be", and then try to relieve the infant's distress. The infant now has had an experience that what had felt intolerable can be tolerated and contained by their caregiver. Over time, experiences such as these will help the infant to develop an internal trust that distressing emotions, while upsetting in the moment, can be understood and be relieved. With growing maturity, this will help them to deal with future adverse experiences in an emotionally responsive and containing way and to develop emotional resilience. However, if an infant repeatedly experiences that their distress does not get acknowledged and contained by another mind, if the caregivers are, for whatever reason, unable to "take in" and feel the infant's distress without themselves getting overwhelmed by it, then the infant is left with the perception that such feelings are, indeed, intolerable. The infant's psyche then has to find some extreme form of coping—for example, by completely cutting off from emotions. In the longer term this could develop into an unhealthy pattern of managing feelings that can have an impact on the person's future mental health.

Bick (1968) formulated a model of containment using the skin as a metaphor. She describes how being contained by its caregiver—being held and looked after emotionally—is experienced by the baby as a skin: such containment holds the infant and its whole personality together, just as one's body feels being held together by one's skin. Bick describes how infringements of this sense of being held together can leave the infant exposed to terrifying fears, such as falling forever or breaking into bits. Skin provides a boundary between self and others, holding one together psychologically. Invasive medical treatments physically break through this protective containing layer. "[W]hen this boundary is constantly being pierced, as it must be in cancer treatment, there can be no sense of being intact, or even safe, in one's own skin" (Hall, 2003, p. 120). The parents might be too traumatized themselves to be able to provide this emotional containment. Hence, the usual protective, containing layers around the infant are doubly invaded, their physical skin being penetrated as well as the "psychic skin" of the caregiver's containing function not being available.

Going through cancer and its treatment at a young age can have a huge impact on a child's future life in terms of physical late effects, but it also might affect their mental health. Even though they might not have conscious memories of this time period, yet their internal, emotional life might be significantly affected. Their psychological coping mechanisms might have been developed in certain ways due to this early traumatic experience. Their perception and expectations of the world, of their relationship to themselves and to others, might have been influenced in ways that are not in their conscious awareness.

Break in the continuation of one's narrative

The diagnosis of cancer and the period following dislocation from ordinary life can bring about a kind of shell shock, engendering trauma: it "plunges the normal individual into the abnormal world of the hospital"

(Goldie & Desmarais, 2005, p. 9). For infants, children, and adolescents diagnosed with cancer, the disruption of ordinary life occurs at the major period of development. Cancer and its treatment can have direct effects on physical and cognitive development, sometimes leaving the person with a disability or disfigurement, and can affect growth and fertility. It can slow, hinder, or even reverse development. For the childhood cancer survivor growing up, the ordinary developmental struggle of moving into independence and the responsibilities of adulthood can be a tricky business.

Hasina

Moving out from her parents' home in order to go to university is a frightening thought for Hasina. She finds any responsibility a burden and is scared of independence. Exploring this in more depth we come to understand that on a deeper level "detaching" has a particular significance to her. She had managed to get through and complied with the long and arduous cancer treatment. But when she reached the end of the treatment, instead of feeling elated, it brought her to the edge of deep despair, and she wanted to end her life. "I have been lying there in hospital, chemo going in, attached to a tube, for so long"; when she got "detached" from the tubes and from the hospital, it put her in touch with primitive fears of being pushed out into the wide world and abandoned, like a helpless infant left to her own devices.

Hasina had a double dependency: one bad (the treatment), one good (the comfort of protection from the outside world). Being looked after in such an all-encompassing way felt reassuring, and even the routines of the hospital could feel comforting. Young people who have spent long periods in hospital often describe how the nursing team has become like a family to them.

Chloe

Chloe often thinks back to when she was younger. So much reminds her, and certain smells make her feel very distressed. However, she also feels drawn to the memories. There is something comforting about them. The experience has been so much part of her life, and when she thinks back, she feels more real and alive. She worries telling me this, as if afraid that by talking about it the memories could be taken away from her. They are so much part of her life.

Chloe seems to have a private and intimate relationship with her memories, and she fears that someone might change this relationship she has with that part of herself, afraid of losing these formative parts of her life.

Independence can feel very scary for the young person as well as for their parents, who, having fought for their child's survival, might hold on to them just a bit tighter than they might have done without this experience. The move into adulthood seems to be particularly difficult for some of the young people who have had childhood cancer. It is often at this transitional stage that it becomes a trigger point: most of the referrals to our team of young people with late effects come at the age of emerging adulthood. During the treatment their ordinary life had been disrupted: periods of missing school, missing activities and social events, sometimes for months and even years. In the work with young people undergoing cancer treatment, feeling excluded from their peer group is a common narrative. While they are stuck in hospital, their peers continue to live their ordinary lives. This sense of being stuck can continue long beyond the treatment and is often present, whether or not the person consciously remembers the period of when they had been treated. Times of transitions, such as leaving school, seem particularly pertinent, resonating with feelings of being left behind while their peers are moving on with their lives.

Deepak

Deepak describes how "before cancer" he was a happy-go-lucky child who dreamed of becoming a professional footballer. Those dreams have long disappeared. The year in hospital changed everything. After his operation, he could no longer play football. "Before cancer" he had connected with his friends through sports and other activities. When he came back, he became identified as "the kid with cancer". He had to start afresh again, making new friends, catching up with school work, which took a lot of energy. In secondary school he did not tell anyone, trying to put it all behind him. But that, in turn, makes him feel that there is an important part of his life that even his closest friends do not know about—as if his narrative, his life story, is broken at that point in time, and he is two different people: a Deepak of "before", and a different Deepak of "after". Since finishing school, he has been feeling lost, and that he does not have the energy to re-start his life yet again: "I am 21 years and don't know where to go from here".

Adolescence brings with it huge emotional upheaval. The adolescent is faced with endocrine, physical, psychological, and neurological changes, as well as having to negotiate wider social and cultural pressures (Waddell, 2018). Searching for answers to the question, "who am I?", is just one aspect. Adolescents might try out different identities in the process of finding a sense of who they are, what they think and feel, how they are different from their parents. For someone who has had childhood cancer, developing a sense of an integrated self is even more complicated and can feel, like Deepak did, that their sense of "continuity-of-being" (Winnicott, 1960) has a break in it, with gaps or a time period that is felt to be completely different from the rest of their lives. To be faced with issues of survival and death at such a young age can prematurely break one's trust in the certainty of life, one's faith of the future.

Anna

Anna describes feeling jealous of her friend who is getting all excited about a boy she has met. Anna herself cannot get excited about such ordinary things. Everything she does brings up questions such as, "What's the point of this?" Having been in touch with death, both her own and of other children she was with on the ward, she "knows" there is no point in struggling to make herself a future, when it can all be taken away in a heartbeat. Anna tells me she wishes she could make her mind "un-know" what she knows. She wishes to be ignorant, to go back to the time where she was carefree and innocent about "the facts of life", a pre-cancer childhood which, in her mind, she imbues with being carefree, happy, and full of life.

Childhood cancer has a huge impact on the whole family's life, reverberating far into the future. Their whole biographical narrative might get separated into a "before" and an "after".

Baby Tamsin

Mother of baby Tamsin feels tormented by her thoughts about her child. She cannot get rid of her sense that the toddler in front of her is not the same child as the baby she used to have before the cancer diagnosis and treatment. In her mind they are two different children, and she feels so disconnected from her memories of before the diagnosis that those memories seem to belong to someone else.

For a parent, their child's cancer treatment can also be associated with the sense that their life's narrative has come to a break, that as a family they have shifted onto another track from the rest of the word, moving along on a different course and in a different direction from the world they had known up to this point:

Ms Kahn

Ms Kahn, with her 8-year old going through a long treatment, tells me how she struggles to stay connected to her family and friends. She says she feels angry when they try to reassure her and say: "it'll be alright in the end". Ms Khan says that they don't know that, they have no idea what it's like in her position. When here in the hospital, Ms Kahn feels at home, while also thinking that this is wrong, she shouldn't be feeling like that. But here in the hospital she gets her experience acknowledged, unlike "out there", when she feels so different from anyone else. While knowing she needs her friends, she isolates herself from them. She says she just gets so annoyed about seeing her friends' lives and their "mundane preoccupations".

Ms Kahn's is not an uncommon experience, and many families with a child who has cancer can feel isolated and different from other people who are not in the same situation. It can be very helpful to meet other families within the paediatric cancer services. Within the hospital environment, their experience makes sense, while outside, where people go about their ordinary lives, the feeling of being different becomes starker.

For a young person who does not remember the time when they had cancer, the sense of being disconnected from one's own history can be even more pronounced. While they "know" on an emotional-sense level about the gravity of their history, this knowledge does not have any conscious memories to connect with. It is other people, such as parents and medical staff, who hold the factual information of what happened to them, and this can cause a feeling of not owning one's own history and experience.

Keith

Keith feels different from his fellow teens. They don't know that he had cancer as an infant, and he does not want them to know. When he comes to our teenage and young adult services, seeing other young people who come for follow-ups or who are on active treatment, he also feels different from them. He cannot identify with being someone who had cancer, because he has no memories of this. All he knows is what his parent and the medical staff in the follow-up clinic have told him. He does not feel that this is his experience and his history. He feels disconnected from his past and struggles to find an identity.

In our appointment, Keith claims that he is fine. He says that because he doesn't remember anything, it doesn't affect him. Yet the narrative he tells me is full of inexplicable problems. He feels "messed-up", and not knowing what's caused it makes him at times overwhelmed by a sense of despair. At another appointment, he tells me that he does have memories, which, he says, is weird, as he knows they cannot be memories. Just like in a dream, he sees himself in them. He feels troubled by these memories or, rather, fragments of imagined experiences. They are not objective reality, he says. It's confusing. He does not want to check out these memories with his parents, because he knows his "memories" will be different from those of his parents. Keith seems frightened that his parents' memories might negate his own—as if only one truth, one reality, is allowed to exist. He wishes to have something of his own.

The sense of gaps in one's own historical narrative is a very common experience for the medical staff running the Late Effects Clinic. It is often very emotional for the patient attending their first follow-up appointment as an adult. They are given the medical information regarding the treatment that they had had, which sometimes up to this point they had never seen, because when they were children this was held by their parents or carers. At the Late Effects Clinic appointment they are being given information about potential longer-term side effects of the treatment that they had— such as potential infertility and increased risk of future health problems— information that can be very hard to bear. The enormity of this realization, that something that happened to them as a child is still having an impact on their present and future lives, can be difficult to take in. At the same time, it is often experienced as very helpful to hear their medical history. It might help with putting together disconnected fragments of memories or sense impressions. These appointments are so important: being treated as an adult, in their own right, about their medical history can give the young person a sense of ownership over their own history.

Paradoxes

With invasive medical treatments, at the level of emotional experience, there is an inherent confusion between the good and the bad. Chemo- and radiotherapy are, at the same time, both toxic to health and agents to better health. One is being poisoned and healed at the same time and by the same substance. It is very tricky for the psyche to process and make sense of this inherent paradox. The good nurse caring for you while you were unwell in hospital is also the "bad" nurse who gave you injections; the "good" doctor who gave you life-saving treatment is also the "bad" doctor who gave you treatment that made you feel very ill. This is compounded when, as is often the case depending on the cancer and its location, the child might not actually have felt ill before the cancer was diagnosed.

In her study on a paediatric haematology and oncology ward, Hall (2003) gives a vivid account of the dichotomy that is part of the nurse's role. This role alternates between giving invasive and painful treatment on the one hand, and being the one who looks after and cares for the ill child on the other. During the initial phase, the child has to undergo invasive procedures, delivered by nurses who, at this point, do not yet know the child. Hall describes this as external trauma. Once treatment such as chemotherapy has stabilized and healthy cells are recovering, the child gets sick from the side-effects of the medication, and the nurses try to alleviate distressing symptoms that are coming from the child's own body. This is an internal trauma. "During internal trauma the child literally must trust us with its life, having previously, during external trauma, often fought against us" (Hall, 2003, p. 121).

When being given invasive procedures, the traumatic experiences are perceived as coming from outside oneself, and the people giving the treatment can be felt as the "persecutors". In the post-chemotherapy phase, traumatic experiences are perceived as coming from one's own insides, from one's body, and the body can come to feel like the enemy. In addition, being dependent and feeling unwell increases one's sense of vulnerability. "The repeated cycles of chemo, nausea, vomiting and diarrhoea could be likened to infantile experiences of being fed, being sick and defecating" (Hall, 2003, pp. 121–122). This experience might leave a confluence in the deeper layers of the mind that associates being helped and looked after with getting sick and with intrusive experiences.

Verity

Verity, a successful and social young woman, tells me of an underlying mistrust of people. For years she has not allowed anyone to come close to her. She feels confused by this and questions if there is something wrong with her. She has been reluctant to receive any help, and in the early phases of our work she was suspicious and denigrating about the psychotherapy. Eventually we were able to think about this, and she made the connection with the medical interventions she had had as a child as part of her cancer treatment. The main thing she remembers about "that time" is fear—fear of being given needles, fear of vomiting, fear of not knowing what is going to happen. She was terrified of losing her hair and was terrified of dying. Her overriding sense was one of "being done to". The various catheters that she had to have to get medication administered or blood taken from made her feel that "I have been stabbed everywhere in my body". She did not feel prepared for it all and felt utterly confused about what was going on. She recounts an incident of someone holding her down to pull out a tube that was down her nose. She thinks it was her parents who were holding her down. Maybe this was even her parents. In our appointments, she often tells me: "I don't blame them." She appreciates what her parents and the medical staff had done for her, and she worries about the other kind of thoughts and feelings, such as that those she rationally trusted had done this to her.

Knowing logically that the intrusive treatment was "for your own good", it becomes hard to acknowledge and feel okay about having feelings of anger and blame. Yet the danger is to turn this anger onto oneself instead and being left with guilt and self-criticism.

> In our appointments Verity realizes a connection between this childhood experience and what happened to her as a teenager, where she "went off the rails", as she describes it. She would abuse her body through toxic amounts of alcohol, and she self-harmed by cutting her arms. At least it was she herself who was now in control of doing the "being done to". She doesn't self-harm anymore. She does like getting tattoos and proudly shows me some of these. Her tattoos have caused some frustration within the medical staff in follow-up appointments, where she refuses to have blood tests because of her fear of needles. To her this feels very different: in the tattoo parlour she feels in charge of what is going to happen to her body.

The volatility of adolescence in itself, with endocrine changes, brain development, and having to cope with changes in one's body, can trigger impulsive and risk-seeking behaviours. Emotional conflicts can become expressed through how the adolescent sees and treats their body. Infantile and childhood experiences of their bodies "being done to" through medical treatment might create an addition layer of pressure on an adolescent psyche. Pubertal bodily changes can in themselves be unsettling for anyone; for the adolescent who had cancer, pubertal changes might unconsciously resonate with their past experience of body changes due to the cancer or treatment (such as losing hair, becoming pale, steroid-induced puffiness). The relationship to one's own body might have been affected, for example, by feelings of their body having failed them. In addition, adolescence might be the time the person becomes more aware of any differences in their bodies due to the cancer or treatment such as scars, surgery, or reduced growth rate.

Feelings of powerlessness and helplessness against the cancer and during treatment might be coped with through a psychological mechanism whereby the passive state is turned into an active one (A. Freud, 1936), like Verity, who takes charge when she gets tattoos done. The confluence of being looked after and being given stuff that hurts, as described earlier, particularly in circumstances where a hospital stay became a significant part of someone's childhood, might set up a psychological mechanism whereby the person unconsciously seeks out such "familiar" stimulation.

Deepak

Deepak does not want to follow his siblings and peers and go into the "boring and bland" life of a 9–5 job, a spouse, and kids. As a child, his peers found him interesting because he had cancer. But now he just feels different from his peer group. He likes engaging in dangerous sports and constantly strives for excitement. Having survived when other children on the ward did not makes him feel indestructible, like a weed that cannot be killed off. When not doing exciting things, he feels dead.

Earlier I referred to how the traumatic experience can impact on a parent's ability to emotionally contain the child's distress. In addition to the huge distress of the cancer diagnosis and fear for the child's survival, parents are faced with an impossible dilemma that the paradox of the treatment brings. The parent has to formally consent, to witness, and often actively coerce their child to undergo painful procedures, or soothe them while medical staff undertake procedures that the child is scared of. What a dilemma to have to face: in order to protect your child, you have to cause her or him pain. In a moving account of observing an infant who at 8 months old developed a cancer in his eye, Davies (2003) describes how the infant's parents tried not to think about the child's vulnerability and, instead, just focused on his resilience. While this might be a way to cope with having to "hand over" one's child to be hurt by invasive and painful treatments, the focus on strengths and positives fails to acknowledge the child's distress. The child may be left with the sense that their distress is not seen, that their experiences are not valid, that their reality is different from the other's reality. In the longer term, this may create a critical evaluation concerning one's feelings ('I shouldn't feel upset over this") or even a sense of disconnection from their own bodily and emotional experience.

Kieron

Throughout his adolescence and as far back as he remembers, Kieron has been feeling like an automaton. He functions well in school and at home, but he feels empty inside. Apart from wanting to be successful, he does not really care about anything. He never feels angry, but neither does he feel joy or connection with others.

Kieron feels like an automaton; Deepak strives for excitement; neither is connected to any feelings of vulnerability, sadness, anger, or other nuances that make up our emotional lives.

Conclusion

Research studies indicate that while many survivors of childhood cancer adjust well after treatment and lead normal and fulfilling lives, there are some who show significant psychological difficulties, such as low self-esteem, anxiety, depression, withdrawal, post-traumatic stress syndrome, intrusive thoughts, drug misuse, increased anxiety, somatic complaints, and disturbances in body image, even years following treatment and often increasing over time (Eilertsen, Rannestad, Indredavik, & Vik, 2011; Fidler et al., 2015; Friend, Feltbower, Hughes, Dye, & Glaser, 2018; Servitzoglou, Papadatou, Tsiantis, & Vasilatou-Kosmidis, 2008; Wiener et al., 2006). Longer-term psychological health seems particularly affected for people who had cancer treatment when they were very young. Their limited cognitive and psychosocial abilities make it more difficult to cope with the traumatic effects of treatment (Servitzoglou et al., 2008). All these studies advocate ongoing routine psychological assessments and availability of support services for this population across the lifespan.

The impact on a family of childhood cancer is immense and often traumatic. Undergoing invasive and toxic but life-saving treatment brings emotional pressures and paradoxes that are challenging to negotiate and make sense of. The impact on a mind still young and immature is particular severe. It can reverberate inside the psyche in years to come and leave the adult survivor of childhood cancer with thoughts, fantasies, and emotional states that seem unconnected to their present lives and that they cannot make sense of. Exploring themes from my clinical work with young people who have had childhood cancer and with parents who have a child undergoing cancer treatment, I have found that on the level of emotional experience both parent and child are impacted by similar or complementary traumas and paradoxes.

Acknowledgement

I am grateful to Susan Mehta and Alison Webb, Clinical Nurse Specialists in Late Effects, for the description of the Late Effects Clinic.

CHAPTER SEVEN

Hope and despair in the face of life-threatening disease

Claudia Henry

La Speranza 'e l'ultima a morire.

[Italian saying: "Hope is the last thing to die".]

The famous ancient Greek myth of Pandora's Box offers an apt metaphor for the main themes of this chapter. Pandora and her husband, Epimetheus, are asked by the god Mercury to look after a magnificent-looking box, on condition that the box must never be opened. Pandora is curious about what lies hidden inside, imagining it to hold beautiful jewels and gold. One day, after wishing so often to look inside, Pandora's curiosity gets the better of her:

> ... and she grabbed the box and pulled at the gold cord and knots. But to her surprise when she lifted the heavy lid there was no gleam of gold or treasure, and not one beautiful dress! Instead, the gods had packed the box full of all the terrible evils they could think of. Out of the box poured disease, misery and death, all shaped like tiny buzzing moths. The creatures stung Pandora over and over again and she slammed the lid shut. Epimetheus ran into the room to see why she was crying in pain. Pandora could still hear a voice calling to her from the box, pleading with her to be let out. Epimetheus agreed that nothing inside the box could be worse than the horrors that had already been released, so they opened the lid once more. All that remained in

DOI: 10.4324/9781003325475-8

the box was Hope. It fluttered from the box like a beautiful dragonfly, touching the wounds created by the evil creatures, and healing them. Even though Pandora had released pain and suffering upon the world, she had also allowed Hope to follow them.

[*The Guardian*, 1 July 2003]

The Italian saying quoted above, along with this Greek myth, illustrates aptly ideas relating to the subject under discussion—namely how, in the midst of "disease, misery, and death", we help our patients and ourselves to sustain hope, in whatever form it may manifest itself.

In this chapter I explore some of the multitude of emotions we encounter in young people we work with, who have experienced a cancer diagnosis. I reflect on how these impact on them and their families, but also on how we, as clinicians, can find ways to understand the impact the work has on us.

Much has been written about working with post-traumatic stress, but a great deal of our work takes place with young people who are actually in the grip of trauma in the here and now and, as such, may require a rather different response. A consideration of this is of particular pertinence to our work and one of the main areas I explore. We do not always work with *post-traumatic states of mind* but, often, *in the midst of traumatic states of mind*. This experience can be very different from one of working with the consequences of trauma at a later stage—something that we do encounter, but more in our work with patients' post-treatment.

Often what we hear being spoken or thought about is in the realms of life and death: fear, despair, and hope within the context of a trauma being lived in that moment.

It is hard, if not impossible, to make emotional sense of the death of or the threat of death in a child or a young person. When working with young patients facing their mortality in such a shocking way, we often bear witness to the limits of feelings that can be endured. We work with these feelings in these young people and children but also, of course, in the parents and families who travel alongside them.

I am reminded of the mother of a patient who spoke of "knowing it for" her daughter when her daughter was in the grip of despair following a cancer diagnosis. The "it" this mother spoke of, and which she was making a huge effort to hold onto, was the hope that, in the pain of diagnosis, the patient had understandably lost sight of. The patient was gripped by shock and fear, and only the words of her mother holding onto some realistic hope could allow her some moments of solace.

As professionals, we cannot give answers to the why, but we can try to at least bear something of the enormous unspeakable burden being carried by the parent or child, or to "know it" for them, be it despair or hope, when they cannot access it. Really listening in this way is painful; I think we are often tempted just to *hear*. Being able to really stay with what is being said and to hold and take in the deeply painful feelings that we are listening to can be a big challenge. As professionals in this area, we are asked to hear, listen, and bear what is at times the unthinkable or the un-hearable, in a society where death and dying are not often discussed.

Communications can come in many different ways and at any time. I am reminded in this work of the experience of a parent with a young child who might ask a pertinent question at any time or place, then move quickly onto something else. They have given their parent the question but do not necessarily need the answer right there and then. It can leave one unsteady, feeling it needs addressing *now*, but the young people, children, and parents we see can only be ready to think about such devastatingly painful feelings *as and when* they are ready to do so.

As clinicians in this field, this is maybe one of the most complicated but important areas when thinking about our responses to our patients.

I recall a mother who was offered support after her daughter had received a devastating prognosis. Again and again the mother politely declined, saying she was "ok, thank you" and did not need help. With some patients this would be a clearly heard message, but with this mother, who was very isolated, there was a strong, repeated endeavour from the medical team to offer her support. Her clinician kept returning, "just to say hello". Sometimes they would accidentally cross each other in other parts of the hospital or outside—and so it went on. Some four months later, her daughter had undergone surgery, and although she still had a poor prognosis, she was recovering as well as could be hoped in the circumstances. On one visit, the mother began opening up to the clinician about their plight, and movingly telling her clinician how important her persistence had been. The mother described how scared she was of the unbearable reality she was facing. The clinician's persistence, returning over and over, somehow enabled the mother to trust that her feelings would not be "too much" and that the clinician could bear to hear her worst fears for what might befall her daughter.

In time it becomes clear that each person has their own tempo to begin thinking about what is, for many, one of the most challenging of areas: that of mortality. Ward staff often speak of a young person asking them suddenly in the middle of the night, seemingly out of nowhere, if they are going to die.

There is a shamanic belief that when a person experiences trauma, a part of themselves leaves their body, so as to protect it until a time when they are able to integrate it back into their being. At that point they physically go and look for that part of themselves and bring it back. The belief implies that at that time, the feelings associated with the trauma will be no less intense than when they were first experienced, but there will then be the emotional capacity to manage the intensity of the feelings better and to integrate them back into the self.

As clinicians in this field of work, we need to be sensitive to the times when the *in-trauma* state is too painful to manage and so cannot be thought about, and times when—even if only for a short moment—it can.

Another mother was seen for some time when her daughter went through many rounds of treatment, as still the cancer kept returning. I think she knew that her daughter's life expectancy was limited. Her knowledge of this came into her accounts of how they were all managing, but often needed to be listened out for by the clinician, as otherwise it could become almost lost in her account. When she could voice it, the clinician would repeat the mother's sentence, using her words, until a time when the moments of acknowledgment could be extended for longer, and the clinician could bear witness to the unbearable loss the mother knew would soon befall her and the family.

Two areas of feeling I have observed are often present when thoughts turn to mortality are those of the title of this chapter: *hope* and *despair*. There are, of course, a myriad other feelings that come to the fore, but it is these two aspects of experience I primarily explore.

Despair can show itself in numerous ways, from screaming, to anger, to quiet withdrawal, and at times lead to reactive depression. Hope can be real or imaginary. It can be a hope for something one would expect, such as to be cured or not to have a re-occurrence or spread of the cancer. It can also be a hope for something small but *so* important: the hope to have a good day or hour. "*Hope is the last to die.*"

These feelings can be experienced by all working with these young people. It is not uncommon to feel overwhelmed and despairing, feeling that not enough is being done to make things better for a young person, child, or family, and a feeling of unmet need can sometimes permeate wards. Maybe that feeling is nothing but the unmet need of the acknowledgement of a reality that it is not always possible to save a life, that restored health is not always achieved, and that even if it is, there is often a long, difficult, and uncertain journey to endure. It is a journey that does not, as with many other health journeys or traumas, have a definite resolution. Once treatment is finished, we know that the emotional and physical fall-out and real risk of re-occurrence or spread does not. There are of course for many also the "late effects" that can emerge as a consequence of treatment, that act as a reminder of their experience.

Alongside despair, however, is the hope, the kindness and humanity, the wish to support, and possibilities of a cure that are what hope is about for many patients.

Feelings of hope and relief when medical treatment has gone well can be felt, alongside despair and feelings of sadness about the trauma that has been endured and the uncertainty it has unearthed around survival and mortality. It is very common to hear young people say, "My treatment is over, I should be happy, but I'm not, I feel so lost" (or alone, or low).

The physical experience is significant here, of course, but also the emotional experience, and it is often the case that the two of them do not run alongside each other hand in hand. It is as though there is a tug of war between body and mind, hope and despair, life and death: a complexity and fluctuation of emotions that is so often described by patients as a "roller-coaster". These feelings can also surface at different junctures.

It is common within the Psych-Oncology Team to meet with patients many years after treatment. This is especially true of young people who were treated as children or infants. Maybe it was the parents who were asking for support at the time. Feelings of hope and despair can resurface or be triggered at times like moving to secondary school or, particularly, leaving education and moving into adulthood. The young person may feel a strong need to have their experience and story heard and in some way integrated, before they can take move into the next chapter of their life.

To illustrate working with feelings of hope and despair, I give two vignettes, one of work with a parent and one with a young person.

When working on open wards or in outpatient settings, there is often not the privacy where feelings may be thought about with patients and their families. Raw emotions may be displayed in a corridor, outside a lift, or by the bedside. One of the challenges is to allow the expression of a rich tapestry of raw emotions in a hospital, where raw emotions can be felt to be threatening, maybe because there are such torrents of them to manage. They are not just seen as a normal response to extraordinary circumstances, as Menzies Lyth (1988) has discussed in her writings. In a hospital there is a thin veil between life and death, illness and health, and within these powerful experiences lies a whole host of feelings.

Amelia and Mary

Mary is a mother in her mid-40s. She has three children. Her eldest daughter, Amelia, who is 12, had a delay to her diagnosis, as the cancer was missed several times. In that time it had spread, and the cancer had advanced. She is being treated, but new symptoms have recently developed, and she has had more tests to investigate these. I have heard in a meeting that the results revealed a further spread of the disease, but Mary and Amelia are yet to hear this news.

In the midst of such painful and complex work we are, as clinicians, also at times in the position of knowing and needing to hold on to knowledge that as yet the family have not been given.

Amelia is at the hospital school when I approach her bedside. We had arranged that I would come at this time, so as to give Mary time to meet with me on her own. I have met Mary on two prior occasions. I have spoken to the nurse, and know that, as yet, they have not seen the doctor to hear the results, but that he could come at any time. Mary is sitting looking into the distance out of the window. As I approach the bedside, I have a familiar feeling of wanting to be elsewhere. This feeling can often envelop a therapist when their patient, or parent, is struggling to allow difficult and as yet unprocessed feelings in mind. This feeling can permeate the whole ward, as it is not a place where patients choose to be. My feeling subsides as I approach Mary. I wonder with her if it might help for us to find a private place to meet. Mary nods. Ward staff help find us a corridor entrance to a side room, where we can close the doors.

The intensity of feelings of hope and despair can come and go from minute to minute in us too, as clinicians. A feeling of dread would be an appropriate description of my wish to not be on the ward. This feeling can, however, quickly be replaced with hope of a meeting that might provide some relief for the patient, even if only the relief of someone having heard their despair as fully as one can.

Mary sits with her shoulders hunched and her fists clenched, seemingly holding herself together as she recounts the deterioration she has noticed in Amelia over the past few weeks, and how urgent tests had been done. She is waiting to hear back from the doctor.

She asks, "Could it be the trauma of it all that is bringing about the changes, rather than the worst-case scenario ... or maybe it's the treatment, the chemotherapy." I perceive her longing for some reassurance, some words of solace. I say that whatever the outcome of the tests, she is letting me know about the "trauma of it all", for Amelia, the family, and, indeed, for her. Mary begins to cry. "I thought I was doing ok" she says, wiping the make-up from under her eyes. I am aware we only have rough hand towels at hand. I want to be able to offer her something soft to wipe her eyes. I say this as I hand her the rough towel she reaches out for, adding that maybe crying is ok as well, but for the time being "ok" for her means not crying.

She nods and smiles through her few tears and says, "Yes, I suppose it is. I am so used to holding it together in front of Amelia, I worry that she worries about me too. I know I hold it together in front of my parents, as they are so sad. I don't want Amelia to feel that she can't be whatever she needs to be in front of me. At least she should be able to have that".

I say it sounds as if there is a feeling of need everywhere, and also an understandable wish for her, as a mother, to be able to protect her daughter. There is so much to be managing. Mary nods and shares her worries with me about one of her other children, who is very distressed, and also about her husband, who is having to care for the children alone at home while she is here with Amelia. I feel that Mary is very able to acknowledge the distress in other family members but is concerned that she needs to be all right, not cry too much, to be strong for her daughter and the others. Now, she feels, is not the time for her to cry.

We often hear parents' understandable wish to protect their children from the full impact of their feelings, but this can equally be seen in the young people, even the very young, who wish to protect their parents from the full impact of their fear or sadness. There is often fear that it would be "too much" for their mother/daughter to know the fullness of their despair. To add to this, children and young people who have cancer can often feel that they are a burden on their families, which would be made worse if their families were fully aware of their emotional and physical suffering. As clinicians, we can often be the person to whom the despair can be voiced and the tears cried.

Psychoanalyst Donald Meltzer (1994) wrote about the modulation of "temperature and distance" in a clinical relationship, and it is important to keep this in mind in our work with our patients and their families living *in traumatic states of mind*. At times only a tissue, preferably a soft one, is needed to wipe tears. Although one can acknowledge that it would be ok to cry—after all, what could be more natural—it is important at times to respect needed defences. The parent/child needs to be enabled to carry on. What we can do is gently hold their hand metaphorically—letting them be our guide, step by step, as to what can at any given moment be borne and what cannot.

As mentioned earlier, we are at times the one holding the knowledge of something positive or alarming about a patient's prognosis. It may also be that patients or families have been told about an alarming prognosis, but in the work with us they move quickly between *knowing* that they or their family member is likely to die and the need to talk about a more hopeful future.

This modulation of *temperature* when working with a possibly dying patient is ever more important, so we can allow space and flexibility to follow them and be where they are in their emotional journey. We may sometimes need to keep in mind their reality, but also allow and share their fantasy of what their life could, or should, have been. I have at times visualized the adult life a young patient describes, even though I know it is unlikely that their wish will be fulfilled.

Sometimes we need to just stand alongside our patients in their fantasy of a life that will not necessarily be lived. The patients need at times to have these dreams heard, so they can face their feelings of loss and grief, however poignant and painful this listening is for the clinician.

Tessa

The parents of Tessa, a 4-year-old child who had a life-limiting disease, spoke about their huge distress as their daughter insisted on speaking about what she would be when she was older. They were finding it devastatingly painful to hear, with their knowledge that their dreams of her future too had been shattered, but sensitively recognized the need their little child was showing for their dream of a future, to at least be heard.

In his story, *The Midnight Gang*, children's author David Walliams (2016) writes about a group of children on a hospital paediatric ward, who in many fantastical ways help each other to live their wish. One child on the ward, Sally, we come to understand, has a terminal cancer diagnosis. She is at times left out of the group's games, as if showing how frightening it can be for people, young and old, to be alongside cancer patients.

This is an important experience we often hear about from our patients, how some friends or family can at times become distant, as an expression of their fear. The hospital team then take on an added role, as people who can and do understand and will not turn away.

In *The Midnight Gang*, the main character, a sensitive young boy called Tom, insists that Sally, too, be given the opportunity to have a wish. The group come to agree, and we learn that her wish is to "live a big beautiful life . . . in just one night". The children, undeterred by Sally's failing health, go about setting up her wish, using hospital props to help her live a big beautiful life, from taking her school exams and driving test, having her first car, to holidays, marriage, children, and grandchildren. Walliams writes that it is all played out to the "unmistakable sound of the world's most famous opera aria, 'Nessun Dorma', and the words 'none shall sleep, none shall sleep, even you o princess, in your cold room, watch the stars that tremble with love and hope'."

As Walliams notes, "The words could have been written for Sally. It was a fitting majestic piece of music to accompany the next few minutes which represented a lifetime" (p. 434).

I was reminded when reading this of times when we are asked to hold onto hope as a way of sharing an experience (as the parents of the little child did) that may not actually ever be able to be lived.

Kate

Kate is an 18-year-old girl. She has had a relapse of her disease, which is now incurable, but for the moment is being kept stable by the treatment she is receiving.

Kate is a vivacious, thoughtful girl who is at college doing GCSEs, as she had to delay her education due to previous treatment. During her first meeting with me, Kate spoke about her future with such certainty and clarity that, at first, I wondered if I had the wrong information about her prognosis. She painted vivid, beautiful pictures of a future with a partner and children, a job she loved, and holidays to places she longed to visit. I understood, however, that my knowledge needed to be put aside. In order for her to feel me as safe enough for her to share her fears and sadness, I needed first to really hear, to really know about the future that she wanted, to see it in all its colours.

Once Kate felt I had really heard her dreams and ideas about her future, she moved quickly on to telling me how important it had been for her to go to a school where no one knew her, so she could decide whom she did and did not tell about her illness. She spoke of how hard it was to know whom to trust, as people appeared so scared when they heard she had cancer. Nevertheless, it was difficult to say nothing, as her friends did not understand why she was so tired, why she could not go out in the evenings as they did. She spoke of missing her social life and doing all the normal things people her age do. I felt close to tears as she recounted this.

I felt that what she needed was for me to just hear her plight and hold her gaze as she told me what she felt—maybe for me to try in some way to contain and hold the full scale of her deep, devastating sense of loss about her future. I think Kate felt heard and listened to, and, as Anna's mother said, "at least she should have that". After some time I could speak of how very hard it was, how she was letting me know that sometimes nothing really felt acceptable, sometimes everything felt wrong and so very unfair.

In the context of work with very ill patients, I think one has to review some ideas about unrealistic hope. Psychoanalyst Anna Potamianou

(1997) writes about unrealistic hopes as a "defensive shield in borderline cases". She maintains that certain types of hope are a way of not living in the present, believing that something better is always to come: "the next book I read, the next session, the next encounter".

Her ideas about postponing life and not living in the present are presented in relation to borderline patients, but, as I have described in the case of Amelia, there are times when, in order to engender a feeling of safety, a similar process occurs for our dying patients that will make a painful reality thinkable about. One may have to bear the pain of really hearing and really "seeing" the hopes and dreams of our patients in all their colours, alongside knowledge of a very different reality. This, then, is one way in which we can share hope with them, while holding onto the reality of their situation waiting for them when they are ready to meet it in their own time.

It is quite common for patients and families to acknowledge eventually that they had been told certain aspects of their prognosis but that, at the time, they were not able to hear them. The Shamanic belief I mentioned suggests that we need to wait until they are ready to think about the trauma they are enduring and to bring it back to mind or, as the Shamans see it, back to their body.

To conclude, I should like explore how we, as a staff group, are able to keep the unbearably sad stories and despair that we witness and the hope that is also part of the work in mind.

As a service, we provide, where possible, various platforms in which staff can consider their experiences. In one such staff work discussion group, which was run fortnightly on a ward, I was always struck by the recurring theme of gratitude and appreciation for life that working in the presence of life and death can bring. In the midst of the despair, there is the hope that, through all the pain one is confronted with, a learning about life can also be nurtured. A little like the patients and families we meet with, however, at times the need for defences in the staff were just as needed, so their work could continue: "a short cry in the toilet and on" was a familiar sentence.

Strong feelings of hope and despair can be felt when a patient who has been on a ward for many weeks and sometimes months and/or had many repeated admissions goes home or to a hospice to die.

Staff get to know their patients very well, and at these times a strong sense of loss can be felt. Poignant memories are often shared, and this is helpful. Although despair may be too strong a word, there is often a deep sense of not having been able to say goodbye, or feelings of regret that a life could not be saved and, at times, disbelief that a vibrant, rich life has been so cruelly cut short. It can be of some solace when staff are informed of the death of a known patient, and some sort of a closure can be had and sometimes spoken about. Ways in which staff are told, however, are varied and the shock and finality of the news never becomes less powerful.

Working *in trauma* requires us to be open to witnessing the moment-by-moment experience of our patients and families as they journey through often shocking, deeply painful experiences.

If we only hope they will get better, we may fail to be alongside them in their despair, yet to acknowledge that they may die may mean we are not able to stay with the hope that they still need. We must thus try to bear witness to the despair and hope as they do, allowing the full range of feeling to be heard.

Memories of many of the patients with whom I worked in the service have left me with immense gratitude and humility that they allowed me to be a part, in some way, of their journey. I am aware that from them, their families and the colleagues I worked with, I learnt life lessons that I will continue to carry with me.

Alongside the *"despair, disease, misery and death"* that can be unleashed from Pandora's Box when there is the threat of a life being cut short, existential lessons are often relayed as being a part of the experience. Within that experience "Hope" may *"flutter from the box like a beautiful dragonfly touching the wounds created . . . and healing them"*, if only for a short while.

CHAPTER EIGHT

Working with families
where a young person is facing death

James McParland, Cristian Pena, & Sara Portnoy

> Grandfather dies, Father dies, Son dies—that is the natural order of things and a blessing for the family.
>
> [Buddhist saying]

How do you summarize the immensity of working with children and young people facing death, we ask ourselves? We decided to reflect together on our work from the Psych-Oncology Team at University College Hospital, and from our work at Life Force, the Community Paediatric Palliative Care Team in North London. Sara and Cristian thought that one way to capture these reflections would be through a conversation. James, who also works across these two teams, heard about this conversation and offered to join in. He thought about Sabine Vermeire's suggestion that if you let only one voice speak, it can become a "new truth", and having only two perspectives might create a dilemma or dichotomy for the reader (Vermeire, 2017). Offering at least three voices creates *polyphony* and opportunities for multiple realities and perspectives to be shared, and this seems appropriate for conversations about death and dying, where there is no *one size fits all* and both expert and local knowledge can be useful.

DOI: 10.4324/9781003325475-9

All that is written in this chapter has been learned on the shoulders of children and young people facing death and of bereaved family members. We honour and thank them.

We sit together on a cold winter's day in Sara's office in North London and wonder where to begin. Death is somehow always a sensitive topic to cover, we conclude, and many people prefer to avoid the topic altogether. Is it because it reminds us of the fragility of our own lives and our own inevitable end? Like the opening quotation of this chapter, is there something so incredibly unnatural about parents losing children that it becomes difficult to even think about how to do this sort of talking? How you might begin?

We decided to start with our own beginnings and journeys into this area.

How did we enter this field of work?

Cristian: Sara, you explained that you entered this field of work gradually. Over the years you worked with children who had more and more serious illnesses, and then you started your present job working as a locum psychologist on a paediatric palliative care team because you were unsure whether you would be able to do this type of work. The joke is that you have now been working with the same team for fifteen years!

Sara: That is true. Cristian what drew you to working in this area?

Cristian: If I am completely honest, I think one of the reasons for wanting to be working in this field is that I was frightened by death, and I had a curiosity or need to understand it and maybe even control it. If I worked in the area, then maybe I could control it, for both my loved ones and myself. I know that sounds ridiculous.

Sara: No, I don't think that is ridiculous. I can only speak from the experience of my father dying since working at Life Force, and I think there was something about knowing more about death and it not being such a taboo that made it easier to talk about death with my father, my family, and other professionals involved in his care.

Cristian: My background was in CAMHS and working at a torture rehabilitation centre for refugees. Despite the fact that the act of torture is horrendous, I could, as a psychologist, somehow hold on to the fact that when I was seeing them, they had their traumas behind them—the future could always be better. Working with people facing death in the future is a completely different scenario. How would I go about working with people facing death? What role would I play as a psychologist?

James: Similarly, I was curious about what we might offer as clinical psychologists in this context due to my previous work experiences. I particularly started to think about liberation psychology ideas, as I had worked with people with different potential constraints to their freedom. I felt personally heartened by the idea that steps towards liberation might be possible when facing the challenge of death, despite significant constraints—physical, emotional, practical, etc. This had begun to emerge through my experience working with young people with chronic health conditions and with children and families in the Psych-Oncology Team who were facing a life-threatening condition. Then an opportunity came up to join Sara on the Life Force Palliative Care Team. Knowing that someone as experienced and knowledgeable as Sara would be supervising the role gave me confidence to tentatively take steps into an area which seemed quite daunting!

Sara: I did have experience and knowledge, lots gained from my own supervisor! But also, we all bring knowledges, both personal and professional, to this work, so I hope you felt able to bring them along too, James.

James: Yes, and you saying that has made me think about another experience I'd had, which was my doctoral thesis. I interviewed older LGB (lesbian, gay, and bisexual) people with dementia and their significant others (McParland & Camic, 2018), considering the intersection of a minority sexuality with a significant neurological condition. The people I spoke with were facing significant losses and threats to their identity through their life-limiting conditions. What I noticed was the importance of their significant relationships, partnerships, and friendships as "safe harbours", allowing them to "weather the storms" that life was bringing. It made me want to work with relationship networks to help galvanize these "shelters" and draw on their possibilities as resourceful systems. I also agree with you both about extending our personal stories about death too. I have certain stories, particularly influenced by my cultural and religious background (Irish, Catholic), but have been afforded the privilege of learning about many more.

Cristian: You are so right. The importance of significant relationships really comes up when working with people facing death. I have seen many young people "weathering the storms" together with others and coping relatively well, while others lamented that their friends have distanced themselves at a moment like this.

Has psychology any role to play when the outcome is inevitable?

Sara: Cristian, you and I talked about how this work requires our *presence*. I think that when people feel really listened to and heard by someone who is able to be *truly present* in that moment non-judgmentally, without thinking about what they are going to say next—I think that can be experienced as similar to the feeling of being loved/truly held in mind and cared for. Vikki Reynolds (2012) asks us to imagine what our work would look like if love were absent. She also draws our attention to being very careful about our language with clients. I wonder whether instead of love we could use a word like doing it with "heart".

It also makes me think about Lee's paper, "Making Now Precious" (Lee, 2013). The title of the paper is helpful in reminding me to stay in the present moment. Although she writes about working with asylum seekers, many of her ideas feel relevant for working with parents whose child is dying. Often I think that it is as much *how* you say the words as the things that you say.

Cristian: This work makes you so humble. You soon realize that it is not about having specific methods up your sleeve, but staying in the present moment and genuinely connecting with the person you are working with is what matters. There is one family that I worked with that I will never forget and that taught me so much. I was asked to help a couple to make an informed decision regarding their daughter. The parents were trying to make an impossible decision about whether to opt for further invasive treatment for their child, which would have an uncertain outcome in terms of her quality of life, or whether to stop treatment, which would lead to their child dying. I had to travel alongside them with humbleness and provide a space for these impossible conversations to take place.

Sara: Keeping in mind the four key themes of relational ethics often holds me steady when I begin these conversations. They are: mutual respect, engagement, embodiment, and environment (Bergum & Dossetor, 2005). As Lee (2013) suggests, these take you beyond the spoken or written word.

James: I feel that one of my other roles in these situations is to bear witness to people's stories and experiences. Denborough's *Narrative Justice and the (Draft) Charter of Story-Telling Rights* (2021) guides me in these conversations—particularly the idea that everyone has the right to have their story understood in the context of what they have been through and "their skills and knowledges of survival respected, honoured and acknowledged" (Article 6). I try to hold a space for parents and young people's stories to be told and understood, which means bringing a genuine curiosity and not making assumptions about how people may feel at any given moment. Even when the outcome may be "inevitable", there are opportunities to hear about how young people or their families respond to this with knowledge and skill; I feel it is important for these responses to be documented. For example, I will create therapeutic documents, such as letters about our sessions, or find other ways to hold onto people's stories, such as helping them to write first person accounts and then thinking with them about who they would like to see it, such as other family members or professionals.

Sara: Yes, narrative therapy ideas inform my conversations, including around acknowledgment, documentation, and making meaning out of such difficult experiences.

James: My other thought was that when I have worked with young people and young adults who are coming to the end of their lives, part of my work has been about supporting them in moving towards preferred directions, despite the constraints of their medical situation (Afuape, 2011)—for example, thinking with young people about how they would like to spend their time in ways informed by their values. This can involve asking questions about their hopes for the next day, week, or month and being curious about whether there are things they would like to talk about or activities they would like to do with those close to them. At other times it has involved more of a supportive advocate role, such as assisting them in asking questions of medical staff which were difficult to put into words during a clinic appointment.

What could you possibly say to a tormented parent whose child is at the end of their lives?

James: I feel it is important to acknowledge this situation really is utterly devastating, difficult to comprehend, and contravenes all of the hopes and expectations of parents. At first, I found it tricky to think about how "hope" could be a part of the conversation in therapy at these times and found myself feeling quite helpless, or worse, useless. Sara, I've found some of our conversations in supervision using Weingarten's (2010) ideas about how "hope" can be a verb and something you "do" together to be very helpful.

Sara: It is a very challenging situation and one which our psychology training does not always allow us to feel prepared for. It brings to mind an experience I had with a parent who was a medical consultant herself. Her eldest daughter was diagnosed with a brain tumour. From the point of diagnosis there was a poor prognosis, because it was staged as a Grade 4 tumour. I had worked with this mother and visited her at home for a number of months while her daughter received treatment, but her condition was deteriorating. One day she was overwhelmed with tears, saying, "Today I have lost hope." This is a family that will always stay with me, because I learnt so much from our conversations. She said, "Don't think that when I was given the diagnosis that my daughter had a Grade 4 tumour, I didn't know what that meant. I have given that diagnosis to patients. I knew my daughter would not survive, but as a parent my job was to hold on to hope. Until today, I have managed that, but I can't do it anymore." I have held onto this idea. So, when doctors are concerned that a parent may not be being realistic about their child's prognosis, I may ask the doctor whether they think it is possible the parent is "holding on to hope" because it is the best way that they know of being with their child in this situation.

Also, Weingarten's (2010) concept of *reasonable hope* has been very helpful in our work. This is the idea that reasonable hope can sit alongside despair and is different from the more traditional sense of hope as something that is alongside "wishes". This has been a more pragmatic sort of hope that parents have been able to discuss alongside distress and despair. There is also an idea, like you say, James, about hope as a verb and something you can do together. This can offer a guide for these difficult conversions in that even when the end is inevitable, there are ways of doing *reasonable hope* together.

James: The story you told is very moving, Sara, and I'm struck both by the idea of what a parent's "job" is in this situation and also how our psychology training might have prepared us for these conversations. I think a surprising aspect—for me, anyway—is that some of the ways I work have not been that different from how I work in other contexts. There seems to be a story that when "death" is mentioned, you cannot use more general ideas, but I think you very much can. For example, I have used ideas informed by solution-focused practice (De Shazer & Berg, 1997), such as asking, "If our talking together today were to offer any sort of usefulness to you right now, what might it involve?", "How would you know that our talking was on the right lines?", or "Where would you be moved to if this had been a helpful conversation?"

I have found that sometimes people want to use the talking time in therapy to discuss more practical aspects of their experiences and possible other parts of their "job" as a parent. For example, parents of children with palliative conditions may want to spend time thinking about and planning their child's funeral. At other times their preference has been to discuss how to talk with the child's siblings about what is happening, or to ask for practical suggestions about how to try and relax or look after themselves, to sustain themselves during this difficult time. Throughout the process of these conversations I am informed by "relational reflexivity" (Burnham, 2005) and check in with clients, through asking, "Is this talking comfortable and useful?" and letting them know it is more than ok, it is welcome to tell me if it is not. Some of the feedback has been that the therapy space can be more "neutral" than such conversations with family or friends, where it can be understandably more charged. I am also guided by Fredman's (1997) ideas of "talking about talking" and not making assumptions about the type of talking that will be helpful to someone at any point but, rather, checking out with them which kinds of talking might be of use.

Cristian: I would agree that things come up that you do not expect. Throughout, I let clients know that I am here, I am listening, that there is no "right" way to feel, and I attempt to validate their emotional experiences.

James: I was also thinking how, alongside curiosity and inviting people to define their own experiences, at points I have found myself "normalizing" emotions. For example, I have shared "pre-bereavement" as a concept that people can experience a profound sense of loss when they are anticipating a bereavement. Parents I have worked with have let me know it was useful to know this was not abnormal or "fatalistic thinking". So sometimes affirming has involved sharing psychological concepts, but doing so in a "light" way, which explicitly invites resistance when something does not fit (Afuape, 2011).

Ideas that have guided us in our work with young people and their families

Sara: One idea that I have found helpful relates to the positioning of a therapist during difficult conversations. Michael White (1997a) proposed that therapists remain "decentred and influential": a position where the client's knowledges are placed in the centre, and the therapist provides the conditions within which their stories can be more richly described. I find I am at risk of taking a "centred and influential" position when I am asked for advice, when I am finding the conversation emotionally demanding, or when the story resonates with me personally.

A conversation that comes to mind is when I met with a father on the hospital ward whose daughter was at the end of her life. He was very distressed, and he asked me, "How do I tell my eldest daughter, who is sitting her finals at university in a month's time, that her little sister is dying?" It so happened that my eldest son was sitting his finals in a month's time, and my thoughts went to "how would I tell Alec that his youngest brother was dying?" I immediately felt overwhelmed by emotion. I stopped, I remembered to breathe and feel my feet on the floor to try and ground myself. It dawned on me: I had not been asked how I would tell my son Alec. My next thought was, "I want to try and help this man. What do the experts say about how to break bad news?" Then Michael White's ideas came to mind. I noticed I had unwittingly centred my emotional self, which had led me to grasp for "expert" knowledge. I wondered whether it might be unhelpful to "centre" my knowledges at this point. Instead, I asked this father to tell me more about his eldest daughter: were there any other occasions where they had held a sensitive conversation, and what had helped make that possible.

This made space for him to let me know that one significant time was when he first told her that her little sister had a diagnosis of cancer. Also, he let me know about the times they had spoken about how the treatment was not shrinking her tumour, and he richly described the words he had used, and where they were sitting, and the expression on his elder daughter's face.

Cristian: You telling that story brings to mind an image for me of very shaky ground. How, if we try to have conversations on this shaky ground, either us as professionals or our clients, it can start to feel unsafe. It makes me think of the idea of structuring a "safe place to stand" before we begin to talk about problem stories, traumas, or challenges, and how we can create that safe place through connecting with an individual's skills, abilities, and intuitive knowledge. When you connected with this father's hard-won knowledge and experience-based skills, a safer ground was created to hold him during this extremely difficult conversation, and it became possible to generate ways forward. You were also able to do the same through giving pause, grounding yourself, and connecting with your own *knowings*.

James: It's making me think, too, about the power of more expert knowledges and discourses, and how it can be easy to be seduced into trying to find one that "fits" and resolves a client's dilemma. I notice I am pulled towards more expert positions when I feel "at sea" or on shaky ground too. I think the certainty they can offer is very appealing! I have, however, found the book *Death Talk* by Glenda Fredman (1997) to be hugely influential and containing, as it presents the idea that there are multiple valuable stories about death and dying. Some of these stories are professional knowledges, whereas others come from families' experiences, their relationships, religion, culture, and broader spirituality. Through remaining curious and decentred, as you describe, Sara, multiple possibilities for useful conversation can open up.

Sara: I remember carrying *Death Talk* around in my bag when out in the community when I first started at Life Force! Also, Cristian, I'm glad you mentioned the concept of a "safe place to stand". Ncube (2006) suggests inviting young people into a "safe place to stand" through hearing about their lives aside from problem stories, before you then begin to think with them about the challenges in their life. She gives the analogy of a crocodile in a river (which represents the problem) and how you want to get onto the riverbank (which represents your skills, abilities, important people, and other sustaining discourses), before you are in a better position to start looking at the crocodile. I think this is often a central intention in our work in this context.

One way of getting to this "riverbank position" is through narrative therapy ideas using the "Beads of Life" approach, which I initially developed for young people with a diagnosis of cancer (for a full description, see Portnoy, Girling, & Fredman, 2016). I begin by getting to know the young person apart from their cancer diagnosis. I ask them about their daily lives, skills, abilities, and qualities, important people and the values they have learned from them, and their backgrounds, including family customs and culture. This includes asking them about what they enjoy when they are not in hospital, or what they enjoyed prior to cancer arriving, and they are invited to choose a bead to represent all of these stories. I dare to ask about their hopes and dreams for the future. If someone is near the end of their life, I would ask them about their hopes for the next week or month and also their hopes for family members or friends. As they choose beads, they tell these stories of their lives. We also offer "Beads of Life" to parents, siblings, and other significant people who are travelling alongside a young person in this situation.

James: For me, this brings to mind the idea of "Hopework" (Moxley-Haegert, 2012), and how, through discussion about special achievements and coping or "survival skills", families engage in this sense of hope as a verb, as something you *do* (Weingarten, 2010). Hopework involves the narrative therapy practice of listening for a "double-storied" account (White, 2007), which acknowledges both suffering *and* foregrounding those special knowledges that are sustaining a family through hardship. I also think it's helpful as "hope" then becomes a discourse sustained among people, rather than an individualized concept, which could make people feel inadequate if they do not readily have access to hope themselves in a particular moment. As psychologists, we join and hopefully assist families and other relationship systems in their *Hopework project*.

Sara: The sense of this being a collective endeavour is an important one with the Beads of Life process. When the young person is telling the stories of their life through beads, we intend to have at least one "witness", as for stories to *live* and *breathe* they need an audience. I ask the witness, who may be a parent, sibling, friend, or a professional, such as a nurse with whom they have a close relationship, to give the young person a bead to represent what they have been touched by or what resonated for them when listening to these stories. It can be very powerful for the young person to have an experience of touching someone else's life in this way. To facilitate talking about the story of hardship, we also invite them to choose beads to represent their medical stories.

Cristian: It's making me think about how a cancer diagnosis really brings so much upheaval and loss to a young person's life, potentially widening the gap between who they thought and wanted to be and who they are able to be in the current circumstances. Many young people I have met with describe and experience periods of resurgent sadness, which Weingarten (2012) terms "chronic sorrow". This non-pathological response to a disruption to their self-narrative has often connected with young people telling me they feel "lost", "directionless" or "numb". It feels important to honour and give space for these stories of loss alongside those of survivorship (Pena & Garcia, 2016). It also reminds me of my work with displaced young people seeking refuge in the Jungle in Calais. They described a similar sense of feeling lost or, at times, "unreal", as their lives were disrupted and in limbo.

James: A particular framework which has helped me conceptualize this state for young people is the "Migration of identity" proposed by Michael White (1995). This suggests that when people experience a break from life as they know it, they experience a process of "separation" as they depart familiar shores and enter a "betwixt and between" period. When a young person is diagnosed with cancer, they experience such a moment of separation as they suddenly move away from what is familiar and known and "cross a threshold" into a different space (Lee, 2020). This includes breaking from familiar structures, such as education or employment, as this is often disrupted, or family life, as they undergo invasive treatments in hospital. The space young people enter could be viewed as a "liminal" space for identity, as they are separated from who they know themselves to be (i.e., a young person without a life-threatening condition), and they may say things like, "My world was turned upside down", "I no longer know who I am", or "It feels like life has been put on pause".

Part of our work involves being alongside young people in this liminal phase, which is extremely discombobulating and uncomfortable, as they lose the sense of grounding offered by normative structures and expectations and they manage the uncertainty of a cancer diagnosis. It makes me think about the importance of bearing witness to these struggles through our presence, facilitating discussion where they put words to their experience, inviting them to share any representative images that come to mind, and also affirming that they are not "going mad" (Lee, 2020). There can also be liberation in some ways as people enter a realm of new possibilities compared to the pre-existing status quo (Lee, 2020). For example, young people have told me that since their diagnosis, they have felt it possible to be more honest about their wants and needs, speak with increased confidence to the adults in their world, experience deeper empathy for those who face struggles in life or have had a realization about what is important to them. Parents and other significant individuals in young people with cancer's lives experience a similar migration of identity as their world changes.

Sara: I have also witnessed young people taking up opportunities to explore new commitments, such as volunteering. We offer the "Beads of Life" to individuals and as a group workshop. Young people who are interested are invited back to join us as "peer trainers" to help facilitate future workshops as consultants by experience. A number of young people, including those with extremely uncertain or palliative prognoses, have joined our workshops as peer trainers. They have offered incredibly rich wisdom, such as hard-earned knowledge about living with cancer, and been an inspiration to other young people.

James: The contributions of these young people and the honouring of their skills of living with cancer makes me think of "reincorporation", which is the concluding stage of "migration of identity" (White, 1997b). Reincorporation involves arriving at a new destination in life and connects with the concept of "rites of passage". Many of the young people we meet will miss out on some of the normative rites of passage that their peers experience. For example, they may see friends progress educationally and take further steps towards independence as they leave the family home, while our young people are derailed, delayed, increasingly dependent on parents, and/or have to readjust their expectations.

I can find myself in a dilemma requiring thoughtful balance. On the one hand, the uncertainty around prognosis for some can limit how much young people feel able to explore possible futures, so it feels important to stay present to their stories of liminality and allowing them to be *seen* in the liminal space (Lee, 2020). On the other hand, I can feel pulled to celebrate and punctuate life for young people who may have had such opportunities constrained due to health, through finding alternative ways to acknowledge their skills of living and new pathways to a sense of reincorporation (McParland, Khan, & Casdagli, 2019). This involves creating opportunities for the new identity stories to be witnessed through "communities of acknowledgment" as young people find ways to *reclaim their lives* from health challenges (White, 1997b).

Sara: A number of different pathways we have travelled towards "reincorporation" are coming to mind: for example, the opportunity for stories to be witnessed in our group workshops, which include a certificate ceremony, where we also invite parents or other significant people in the young person's life to bear witness to their skills and abilities. We have also been fortunate to attend conferences talking about our work where young people have joined us to present our projects, including winning a conference award for their contribution, creating further opportunities for new, preferred identity stories to be affirmed.

Cristian: I have been struck by how powerful it has been for people's preferred identity development when they have had opportunities to "give something back". Many young people have let me know they want to help others and *give back* to the cancer community that has helped them. It also connects to parents, too, who have volunteered their time for charities connected to cancer or bereavement, and I wonder if this is a similar experience of reincorporation as they arrive to new destinations in life? I think again about the sense of people re-evaluating what they want their life to stand for in the wake of such an uprooting experience of a health crisis. Similarly, parents may decide to involve themselves with cancer charities or offer peer support to other parents who have experienced bereavement. I have also met parents who completely re-evaluated their lives and involved themselves in different causes. I met one father who became acutely aware of some of the vast inequality in the city, and he decided to join a charity that worked for equality. It may well have been a way for him to channel the sense of unfairness that he was experiencing as a father of a child facing death. In any case, he met a number of people who gave him hope, and it gave him a sense of meaning and control, beyond the fear and sorrow that he was experiencing.

Sara: What underpins much of our approach is recognizing the possibilities that emerge when you intervene beyond individual therapy. We try to create connections and facilitate opportunities to resist and work against the isolation that a life-threatening condition, such as cancer, can bring to young people, their families, and bereaved individuals after death.

In that way I would conceptualize our focus as broadly systemic, appreciating the role of relationships and networks, alongside therapy which may be individual and offers holding and containment.

James: It makes me think about "personhood", which was a specific concept I explored in my earlier research with people with dementia. Kitwood (1997) suggested that promoting personhood is important to counter a state of "living death" when people are faced with significant losses, such as dementia, or, I would suggest, a life-threatening or palliative condition. The components of personhood are attachment, identity, inclusion, comfort, occupation, and what holds them all together: love. This is a social and relational endeavour; personhood is a status bestowed on someone by others, within the context of social relationships. Through our peer groups and opportunities for family and wider system acknowledgment, we are moving away from seeing psychology as solely "internal work" (Winslade, 2002), finding ways for alternative stories to be interwoven into the lives of others (Morgan, 2000), and trying to do it "with heart", as you beautifully described, Sara.

How have bereavement theories helped you in your work?

Sara: This question once again brings to mind Michael White's ideas about the therapist remaining decentred. It is easy to view well-known theories as *expert* knowledge or even "the truth", and they can then barge in and undermine a bereaved individual's experiences. In my work I have used theories tentatively, usually when a client says something that resonates with one of them and I have a hypothesis that the theory may help make sense of some of the overwhelming emotions that they are experiencing in relation to grief. I would always ask whether the ideas fit for them, so I centre the young person or parent's knowledge of whether they have found the ideas helpful.

Cristian: Is this not the problem with diagnoses altogether? In our work with refugees in Calais, Sara, how many refugees' experiences fit into a diagnosis of PTSD (post-traumatic stress disorder), as expected in mainstream trauma psychology? Pain and suffering extends beyond experiencing particular phases or psychological symptoms in the way manuals describe. People experience their suffering multidimensionally: physically, socially, interpersonally, functionally, and existentially, as well as psychologically (Patel, 2019). I often hear a particular story or expectation that to process their grief, people need to "accept the reality of the loss" (Worden, 2009). I remember a bereaved parent finding this a tremendously provocative idea. They said, "I may be able to function with the understanding that my child has died, but I will never accept that it is ok that she died."

Sara: I think that *acceptance* is a difficult word. Is acceptance about saying that it is ok, or is it about not fighting what cannot be changed? "Accepting the reality of the loss" has been proposed as a *task* of mourning. This fits in that it suggests tasks are *hard work* and in my experience and what I have heard from clients, grief is extremely hard work. However, tasks are also things that can be completed, such as "doing your homework", and accepting the reality of the loss is a task that can take a lifetime. Is it accepted when you lay one less place at the table every mealtime? Or many years later, when your youngest sibling celebrates their wedding, accepting your sibling who died is not able to celebrate with you?

James: One model which I have shared and seems to fit for some bereaved individuals is the dual process model (Stroebe & Schut, 1999). There is a suggestion that people move between two coping processes during bereavement: a loss-oriented process, which involves more of a focus on facing the death *head on*, with all of the associated sadness, existential questioning, and sense of unfairness; and a restoration-oriented process, which includes adjusting to new roles and responsibilities in the aftermath of a death, the completion of day-to-day tasks, and a shifted focus from grief. As people describe how they are experiencing these processes and moving between them, I might share the model. This communicates that this *oscillation* is "normal", and the sense of movement between the two processes seems to offer possibilities for people as they find ways to keep going on with life alongside grief.

Sara: That connects for me with another grief theory that people have told me is a good fit, which involves "growing around grief" (Tonkin, 1996). Parents who have lost children have helped me understand that their grief has not tended to get smaller over time, but they have found that life has expanded around it, with new experiences, and feeling able to notice moments of enjoyment. It seems to fit better, as it acknowledges that grief may never totally disappear and there may be particular times when it becomes more intense, such as around anniversaries, but it may become less dominant in someone's life over time. Our conversations in therapy might be about this process, which does not create a sense of disloyalty to the deceased, whom they forever honour, alongside managing to continue with life.

James: Many of the individuals who I have met with in therapy speak about the person who has died still being a part of their life too: these are important relationships that people want to *honour*, as you described, Sara. "Continuing bonds" is a helpful framework that can create opportunities for people to think about how they might like that relationship to be (Klass & Steffen, 2018). A connected idea from narrative therapy is re-membering conversations (White, 1997a), which involve bringing forth the significant contributions from those who have died to the life of the person that is bereaved. It can also involve asking questions to bring the deceased person more into the present, such as exploring what might the person who has died make of developments in the life of the individual in therapy. These sorts of conversations seem to open up possibilities and ways to live alongside profound grief.

Sara: We also invite families to share special memories at our yearly "Memory Day" for those families that have lost a child who was cared for by the Life Force team, where we celebrate those young people's lives through a creative memory activity.

James: Another guiding principle is trying to remain open-minded and not assume that a professional is the best person to do *death talking* or have conversations about bereavement with. Therapy can be a space to review different ideas, but it may be that the most usefulness emerges in another context—for example, through conversation with other parents who have experienced a similar bereavement.

Is it all about the present moment?

Sara: Cristian, you have told me that when you are about to meet the parents of a child who is dying, you wonder what on earth you could say to make them feel better. Then you are reminded of the present moment and that, in this moment, their child is here: they can still create a precious moment, something they can cherish and remember. This again connects with Lee's (2013) idea of "making now precious" and exploring how this could be possible with families.

Cristian: Yes, and I learnt this through talking with families. One parent told me that living with a child with a life-limiting illness taught her about the present moment, because it was the only safe place to be with her child. The past held bad memories, of difficult diagnoses and hospital appointments. The future is terrifying, as it can bring up thoughts of imagining life without her child. If she could find ways to stay in the moment with her son, she could be more comfortable, because this moment involved caregiving, closeness, and connection.

James: Parents have also spoken to me about wanting to be more in the "now" with their child. Following discussion about a future imagined funeral, we've evaluated the talking: parents often let me know that such conversations have allowed them to momentarily put their worry about this to one side and to focus more on the now. It also feels important to appreciate how challenging the "now" can be, reconnecting with the earlier ideas around an uncertain and uncomfortable "liminal space".

Cristian: It makes me think about when a doctor says that, in their professional opinion, there is nothing more they can do for a child, and any further treatment will only cause pain and suffering. Parents then have to make a decision about treatment based on the doctor's information. I will always remember a father saying to me, "It's all very well, you helping us make this decision, but as a parent, it is impossible for me to say that I don't want my child with me for an extra day."

Sara: It brings to mind the phrase, "Matters of life and death are too onerous, too painful to do alone" (Weingarten, 2000). As professionals, we are offering to bear the unbearable and be a compassionate witness to the chaos of emotions that bereaved or dying people struggle to put into words (Weingarten, 2000). Although our work can involve finding ways to *make now precious* and document responses to challenges, we are also trying to offer a safe place where *any* story can be told. This involves embodying presence and trying to *lean in* to others' stories of distress, as Pennebaker (1997) describes: how suffering people who sense their "listener" is apprehensive about the story they are telling, stop talking.

Cristian: Sometimes the stories we hear might not match up with the stories we are told by other people—for example, a client's understanding of a prognosis not fitting with the medical view I have also heard. I remember working with a mother who let me know how her son was her "whole world". From what the doctors told me, I knew that her son was coming to the end of his life, yet she could not contemplate this. It left me with questions about how much should you do a reality check with parents, and how much should you let them hold onto hope?

James: It makes me think about "denial", which is a story I've heard told about parents who do not seem to be overtly "accepting" a poor prognosis. I like Fredman's (1999) idea that "denial" is a *kind of knowing* that someone is showing in a particular context. An example might be when a parent is talking with a nurse who is administering medication to their child at the end of their life, and they ask questions about whether there could be a different treatment that might help. Fredman suggests that there might be several kinds of knowing, of which "denial" is one, and which are shown in specific contexts of time and relationship. If we hold a view that there might be several types of knowing, we become freer from needing to remove or identify the "cause" of the denial. We are also freer from righting someone with "correct" information but can, instead, explore these different *knowings* and who they show them to, including the sorts of opportunities or challenges they create. For example, the same parent may have had conversations with a faith advisor about ideas surrounding the afterlife, which has alleviated some fear for the future, or they may have spoken in therapy about anticipating a time when their child is released from pain, which they anticipate as a relief, having seen them suffer.

Sara: Although I agree that denial needs to be unpacked, there is another process at play sometimes, which I call "the protection racket". Some of the work we do with families when young people are dying is trying to stop "the protection racket" in its tracks by naming it, speaking about it, and examining its tricks and tactics. I've heard that the protection racket tries to talk parents into not sharing difficult information and also their own more distressing emotions with their child. Also, there are some unhelpful prevailing stories that if a young person wants to know what's wrong, they will ask; however, many young people will pick up if their audience is uncomfortable about telling them, which can be silencing. Similarly, the protection racket talks children into hiding their questions and concerns from parents. When the protection racket gets going, it can cause many misunderstandings and can create emotional distance between children and parents at a time when they are craving closeness and understanding. I lightly explore whether the protection racket might be operating for people in therapy, letting them know it can be a very common presence. This seems to allow people to examine and evaluate its effects and consider alternatives.

James: I think it's also important to acknowledge the sustaining effect in the present of future hopes and dreams, and moving into a future-focused space in therapy also seems to create possibilities, however limiting a prognosis seems. When people have a life-limiting condition, or they are parents of a child with a life-limiting condition, or their child has died, they are in the difficult process of adjusting to the potential for a previously imagined future to become impossible. I would proceed carefully, perhaps inviting feedback on how to phrase questions, such as, "should we talk about 'when' or 'if' you have less side effects and can leave the hospital for some time?" Also, hopes and dreams often have a historical context in which they originated, so I may also explore these stories. Moving between the past, present, and imagined futures in therapy seems to create reflexive loops that open space for new possibilities, beliefs, and stories (Boscolo & Bertrando, 1992).

Working with clients who have a faith

Cristian: When I think about families that I have consulted with who have a religious belief or humanistic belief, I have always found it easier to work with them on some level. I find it gives them a structure and a way to *think about the unthinkable,* such as losing a child, or ways for *making meaning* out of their situation.

James: Yes, Cristian, I also think about what having a faith offers to people. This can often be a way to make sense of their experiences and offers sustenance to their situation. For example, when asking young people with a palliative condition questions like "What effect has having your religious faith had for you?", they have told me, "It helps me to understand this is God's way." Or asking bereaved parents, "What difference has your faith made to how you are living with the loss?", they let me know, "At times it feels impossible, but I know God will send me no suffering I cannot bear, so I keep going."

Sara: I think something that I have learned is that solely knowing a person's religion often tells you little about their unique context, so I have tried to resist making assumptions. I ask questions about their faith, their practices and beliefs. For instance, I remember with a young man who was Muslim, who was feeling so bad that he was experiencing suicidal thoughts, I asked, "What has stopped you taking the actions that you have contemplated?" He answered, "Because I can't, it's against my faith", and the clarity about that, the certainty, in that way it helped. Also, I worked with a young Jewish woman who was dying. She did not describe herself as religious, but she did feel her religion offered her a network of people who would be there for her, so maybe you would describe that as her community. For others, the death of their child has made them question their faith, and this expression of different personal ideas can lead them to feeling or becoming isolated from faith communities.

James: I agree, it is helpful to be open-minded and curious about an individual's meaning-making in relation to religion, as this can involve different and sometimes contrasting stories. Initially, I think I was apprehensive, as when people mention religion or "God", it can feel like a very fixed idea, and I did not want to offend or say the "wrong thing". However, I noticed that for some people the effects of ideas were quite constraining. For example, bereaved parents would talk about religious guidance they had received about needing to "move on" or "reach an acceptance", which they were struggling with and did not seem to fit their emotional experience. The effect of these ideas was that they sometimes felt they were "lacking" in some way, which compounded their feelings of hopelessness.

Sara: I see one of our roles as to help explore and generate a repertoire of stories and possibilities around death (Fredman, 1997). What that means in practice is not avoiding exploring ideas and discourses, evaluating the effects of these for people, and offering an opportunity to explore multiple truths. For example, in many religions there can be more than one story. If I hear that a client is in a dilemma about their emotional response to one religious idea, I might be respectfully curious and say, "I hear that there is one idea from your Imam about this, might someone else have a different idea?" or "Have you ever heard any alternatives to that position?"

James: I think it can be helpful to allow people to express their views on different beliefs. So I might ask something like, "Is that an easy or a difficult religious idea to hold onto?" I think this communicates that all emotional experiences are valid and helps to put words to the dilemmas our clients experience. I like your description, Sara, and would perhaps call this positioning *respectful curiosity*. I also try to foreground spirituality as another context to be curious about, as sometimes the comfort people experience does not fit within traditional religious frameworks. People often talk about "signs" or "messages" they feel are communicated to them by their lost loved ones; I give space, time, and affirmation to these stories too.

How does this work impact us as a therapist and as human beings?

Sara: Undoubtedly it has made me appreciate the "small and the ordinary" in my everyday life. It helps me to be grateful that my three children are healthy, and when they complain about going to school, how fortunate I am that their lives are so complete they can complain about very normal things. It has also helped me go on learning and seeking new ways of being with families, because this type of work was not covered in my training. I am reminded of Vikki Reynolds' idea that we learn our work on the backs of clients, and I have learned so much from the many families that I have travelled alongside (Reynolds, 2011). In fact, everything that is discussed here is learned from the parents and young people I have worked with, as well as the articles and books I have read. And I imagine that those ideas came from the parents and young people those researchers had worked with. It also feels important to mention that learning involves making mistakes; I tread very carefully, sensitively, and thoughtfully, as the mistakes we make are experienced by our clients—as I have witnessed you both also doing, Cristian and James.

Cristian: The work has often led me to question my values. When families have made decisions which may be different from the ones I imagine I might make, it pushes me to remain non-judgemental and try to walk a mile in their shoes. Also, the work challenges me to remain curious and keep asking questions, rather than *knowing* too soon. The not-knowing can be a very uncomfortable place to be, so I have had to learn ways of managing to stay with these feelings (Anderson & Goolishian, 1992).

James: I would agree, Cristian, and it has been important for me to let myself off the hook for knowing all the answers, while also continuing to learn, extend my own repertoire of beliefs and stories about death, and keep my work accountable to those who consult with me through continual feedback conversations. The work also makes you think about your own lives, in particular the spirit of "making now precious", encouraging a personal commitment towards celebrating milestones and creating memories.

How do you continue to work in this field and resist burnout?

Cristian: Sara, you have worked in palliative care and bereavement for fifteen years. How have you managed to do this type of work for so long?

Sara: The support I get from my colleagues on the multidisciplinary team (MDT) and my psychology colleagues have been important factors in sustaining me in this work. The work we do together as an MDT is so much more than the sum of its parts. I very much connect with Vikki Reynolds' concept of "collective sustainability" (Reynolds, 2012). Being part of a team who collectively care helps sustain me and resist burnout. Vikki also reminds us that it is not our clients who create burnout—in fact, our clients usually inspire us. Often it is the injustices that families experience that can lead to a sense of burnout. Alongside the support from my teams, I have been fortunate to have supervision from an inspirational and experienced supervisor, Glenda Fredman, who has enriched my practice through every conversation.

I have also been able to work with families after the death of their child, which has afforded me the opportunity of seeing parents and siblings survive the loss of a child, even witnessing post-traumatic growth for some. It brings to mind a parent I met with before her child died and in the subsequent aftermath. The first time we met after the death, she wept and howled, and it was distressing being in the room with so much pain and emotion. At a session 18 months on, she said, "I have managed to find a place where I can be with my daughter." She talked about trying to find some silent moments every day. She also still experienced distressing images of her daughter at the end of her life, and the experience that these images did not stay helped her manage them better in the moments when they were present. She has not forgotten her daughter or "moved on", but has found a way of living and of being with her daughter who has died.

James: When I reflect on my time with the Life Force team, I also think about the parents who have been bereaved and how they find ways to go on alongside grief. Alongside self-care and use of supervision, I find witnessing their commitment to continuing with life after such a profound loss to be heartening and sustaining to witness. I also think in my clinical practice it has been helpful to release myself from a "more pain, more gain" discourse in relation to the emotions discussed in therapeutic dialogue (Yuen, 2009). While there will be a space held for processing more painful and difficult emotions, I have let go of the expectation that it will always be the type of talking people want to do. There can be space for another idea of "less pain, more gain", when you thread through conversations about hopes, moments of joy, celebrations, and special memories.

Cristian: I agree with you both. Having the support from colleagues, like you, James; being able to show your weaknesses and fears in supervision, as you have allowed me to do, Sara; as well as having the privilege of being invited by clients to witness their journey have all given me strength to work in this field. I have learnt that you cannot tame death, you cannot control the future, but you can stay and try to live the present moment to the fullest. I have learned that from my clients.

James: I have found this conversation to be very generative, as through talking with you both I have been introduced to even more ideas and possibilities for conversations in therapy, which have been presented with the lightness of touch we aspire to embody in therapeutic encounters. I'm glad we've had this opportunity to share our learnings and offer a polyphony of ideas. As we describe, we do not see one "right" way to understand or talk about death and dying, so I hope that our readers join us in curiosity and invite them to reflect on how any of the ideas might fit or be of use to them.

REFERENCES

Afuape, T. (2011). *Power, Resistance and Liberation in Therapy with Survivors of Trauma: To Have Our Hearts Broken*. London: Routledge.

Ahmad, S. S., Reinius, M. A. V., Hatcher, H. M., & Ajithkumar, T. V. (2016). Anticancer chemotherapy in teenagers and young adults: Managing long term side effects. *British Medical Journal, 354*: i4567.

Albritton, K., Caligiuri, M., Anderson, B., & Nichols, C. (2006). *Closing the Gap: Research and Care Imperatives for Adolescents and Young Adults with Cancer*. Report of the Adolescent and Young Adult Oncology Progress Review Group. Bethesda, MD: National Cancer Institute.

Aldiss, S., Fern, L. A., Phillips, R. S., Callaghan, A., Dyker, K., Gravestock, H., et al. (2019). Research priorities for young people with cancer: A UK priority setting partnership with the James Lind Alliance. *BMJ Open, 9* (8).

Anderson, H., & Goolishian, H. (1992). The client is the expert: A not-knowing approach to therapy. In: S. McNamee & K. Gergen (Eds.), *Therapy as Social Construction* (pp. 25–39). London: Sage.

Barnett, M., McDonnell, G., DeRosa, A., Schuler, T., Philip, E., Peterson, L., et al. (2016). Psychosocial outcomes and interventions among cancer survivors diagnosed during adolescence and young adulthood (AYA): A systematic review. *Journal of Cancer Survivorship, 10* (5): 814–831.

Barr, R. D., Ferrari, A., Ries, L., & Whelan, J. (2016). Cancer in adolescents and young adults: A narrative review of the current status and a view of the future. *JAMA Pediatrics, 170* (5): 495–501

Becker, E. (1973). *The Denial of Death*. New York: Free Press.

Behan, C. (2003). *Rescued Speech Poems: Co-authoring Poetry in Narrative Therapy*. Available at: www.narrativeapproaches.com/rescued-speech-poems-co-authoring-poetry-in-narrative-therapy

Benowitz, S. (2000). Children's oncology group looks to increase efficiency, numbers in clinical trials. *Journal of National Cancer Institute, 92*: 1876–1878.

Bergum, V., & Dossetor, J. (2005). *Relational Ethics: The Full Meaning of Respect*. Hagerstown, MD: University Publishing Group.

Bick, E. (1968). The experience of the skin in early object-relations. *International Journal of Psychoanalysis, 49*: 484–486.

Bion, W. R. (1959). Attacks on linking. *International Journal of Psychoanalysis, 30*: 306–315.

Bion, W. R. (1962a). *Learning from Experience*. London: Karnac, 1984.

Bion, W. R. (1962b). The psycho-analytic study of thinking. *International Journal of Psychoanalysis, 43*: 306–310.

Bion, W. R. (1967). *Second Thoughts*. London: Karnac, 1984.

Bleyer, A. (2002). Older adolescents with cancer in North America deficits in outcome and research. *Paediatric Clinics of North America, 49*: 1027–1042.

Bleyer, A., Budd, T., & Montello, M. (2005). Lack of participation of older adolescents and young adults with cancer in clinical trials: Impact in the USA. In: T. O. B. Eden, R. D. Barr, A. Bleyer, & M. Whiteson (Eds.), *Cancer and the Adolescent* (2nd edition, pp. 32–45). Oxford: Blackwell.

Bleyer, A., Morgan, S., & Barr, R. (2006). Proceedings of a workshop: Bridging the gap in care and addressing participation in clinical trials. *Cancer, 107* (7, Suppl.): 1656–1658.

Bleyer, W. A., & Barr, R. D. (2007). *Cancer in Adolescents and Young Adults* (1st edition). Berlin: Springer.

Bleyer, W. A., Tejeda, H., Murphy, S. B., Robison, L. L., Ross, J. A., Pollock, B. H., et al. (1997). National cancer clinical trials: Children have equal access; adolescents do not. *Journal of Adolescent Health, 21* (6): 366–373.

Blomberg, B. (2005). Time, space, and the mind: Psychotherapy with children with autism. In: M. Rhode & D. Houzel (Eds.), *Invisible Boundaries: Psychosis and Autism in Children and Adolescents*. London: Karnac.

Boscolo, L., & Bertrando, P. (1992). The reflexive loop of past, present, and future in systemic therapy and consultation. *Family Process, 31* (2): 119–130.

Bowlby, J. (1979). *The Making and Breaking of Affectional Bonds*. London: Tavistock Publications.

Brennan, J. (2001). Adjustment to cancer—coping or personal transition? *Psycho-Oncology, 10* (1): 1–18.

Brewin, C., Gregory, J., Lipton, M., & Burgess, N. (2010). Intrusive images in psychological disorders: Characteristics, neural mechanisms, and treatment implications. *Psychological Review, 117*: 210–232.

Britton, R. (1981). Re-enactment as an unwitting professional response to family dynamics. In: S. Box, B. Copley, J. Magagna, & E. Moustaki (Eds.), *Psychotherapy with Families: An Analytic Approach* (1st edition). London: Routledge.

Bruce, M., Gumley, D., Isham, L., & Fearon, P. (2011). Post-traumatic stress symptoms in childhood brain tumour survivors and their parents. *Child: Care, Health and Development, 37*: 244–251.

Burnham, J. (2005). Relational reflexivity: A tool for socially constructing therapeutic relationships. In: C. Flaskas, B. Mason, & A. Perlesz (Eds.), *The Space Between: Experience, Context, and Process in the Therapeutic Relationship* (pp. 1–17). London: Karnac.

Cancer Research UK (2021). *Young People's Cancer Statistics.* Available at: https://www.cancerresearchuk.org/health-professional/cancer-statistics/statistics-by-cancer-type/young-peoples-cancers

Carbone, P. (1996). Hodgkin's disease in adolescence: A psychoanalytic approach. *Journal of Child Psychotherapy, 22* (1): 128–142.

Carr, R., Whiteson, M., Edwards, M., & Morgan, S. (2013). Young adult cancer services in the UK: The journey to a national network. *Clinical Medicine, 13* (3): 258–262.

Carter, C., & McGoldrick, M. (1999). *The Expanded Family Life Cycle: Individual, Family and Social Perspectives* (3rd edition). Needham Heights, MA: Allyn & Bacon.

CCLG (2021). *Caring for a Child with Cancer in Developing Countries.* Available at: www.cclg.org.uk/podc/caring-for-a-child-with-cancer-in-developing-countries

Cecchin, G. (1987). Hypothesizing, circularity, and neutrality revisited: An invitation to curiosity. *Family Process, 26*: 405–413.

CLIC Sargent (2013). *No Young Person with Cancer Left Out.* London: Author.

CLIC Sargent (2014). *Coping with Cancer.* London: Author.

CLIC Sargent (2016). *Cancer Costs.* London: Author.

CLIC Sargent (2017). *Hidden Costs: The Mental Health Impact of a Cancer Diagnosis on Young People.* London: Author.

Cooper, M. (2017). *Existential therapies* (2nd edition). London: Sage.

Datta, S. S., Cardona, L., Mahanta, P., Younus, S., & Lax-Pericall, M. T. (2019). Pediatric psycho-oncology: Supporting children with cancer. In: J. M. Rey & A. Martin (Eds.), *Jim Rey's IACAPAP e-Textbook of Child and Adolescent Mental Health.* Geneva: IACAPAP.

Davies, A. (2003). Survival and resilience: The impact of cancer on an infant and his family. *International Journal of Infant Observation, 6* (2): 90–110.

Dein, S. (2004). Explanatory models of and attitudes towards cancer in different cultures. *Lancet Oncology, 5* (2): 119–124.

Denborough, D. (2021). *Narrative Justice and the (Draft) Charter of Story-Telling Rights.* Available at: https://dulwichcentre.com.au/charter-of-story-telling-rights

De Shazer, S., & Berg, I. K. (1997). "What works?" Remarks on research aspects of solution-focused brief therapy. *Journal of Family Therapy, 19* (2): 121–124.

Dommett, R. M., Redaniel, M. T., Stevens, M. C. G., Hamilton, W., & Martin, R. M. (2013). Features of cancer in teenagers and young adults in primary care: A population-based nested case–control study. *British Journal of Cancer, 108:* 2329–2333.

Eilertsen, M.-E. B., Rannestad, T., Indredavik, M. S., & Vik, T. (2011). Psychosocial health in children and adolescents surviving cancer. *Scandinavian Journal of Caring Sciences, 25:* 725–734.

Emanuel, R., Colloms, A., Mendelsohn, A., Muller, H., & Testa, R. (1990). Psychotherapy with hospitalized children with leukaemia: Is it possible? *Journal of Child Psychotherapy, 16* (2): 21–37.

Fann, J., & Sexton, J. (2015). Collaborative psychosocial oncology care models. In: J. C. Holland, W. S. Breibart, P. B. Jacobson, M. J. Loscalzo, R. McCorkle, & P. N. Butow (Eds.), *Psycho-Oncology, Third Edition.* London: Oxford University Press.

Fern, L. A., Birch, R., Whelan, J., Cooke, M., & Sutton, S. (2013). Why can't we improve the timeliness of cancer diagnosis in children, teenagers, and young adults? *British Medical Journal, 347:* f6493.

Fern, L. A., & Whelan, J. (2018). Cancer research and AYA. In: J. Chisholm, R. Hough, & L. Soanes (Eds.), *A Practical Approach to the Care of Adolescents and Young Adults with Cancer* (pp. 19–35). Cham, Switzerland: Springer.

Fidler, M., Ziff, O., Wang, S., Cave, J., Janardhanan, P., Winter, D. L., et al. (2015). Aspects of mental health dysfunction among survivors of childhood cancer. *British Journal of Cancer, 113* (7): 1121–1132.

Fisher, J. (2017). *Healing the Fragmented Selves of Trauma Survivors: Overcoming Internal Self-Alienation.* New York: Routledge.

Flynn, D. (2000). Adolescence. In: I. Wise (Ed.), *Adolescence* (pp. 67–83). London: Karnac.

Fredman, G. (1997). *Death Talk: Conversations with Children and Families.* London: Karnac.

Fredman, G. (1999). Denial: a sort of knowing: Conversations about death and dying. *Contexts, 42:* 25–27.

Fredman, G., & Dalal, C. (1998). Ending discourses: Implications for relationships and action in therapy. *Human Systems: The Journal of Systemic Management and Consultation, 9* (1): 1–13; *22* (2): 418–433.

Fredman, G., & Rapaport, P. (2010). How do we begin? Working with older people and their significant systems. In: G. Fredman, E. Anderson, & J. Stott (Eds.), *Being with Older People: A Systemic Approach.* London: Karnac.

Freud, A. (1936). *The Ego and the Mechanisms of Defence.* London: Routledge, 1993.

Freud, S. (1920g). *Beyond the Pleasure Principle. Standard Edition,* 18.

Freud, S. (1926d). *Inhibitions, Symptoms and Anxiety. Standard Edition,* 20.

Friend, A. J., Feltbower, R. G., Hughes, E. J., Dye, K. P., & Glaser, A. W. (2018). Mental health of long-term survivors of childhood and young adult cancer: A systematic review. *International Journal of Cancer, 143*: 1279–1286.

Garland, C. (2003). *Understanding Trauma: A Psychoanalytical Approach.* London: Karnac.

Glaser, S., Knowles, K., & Damaskos, P. (2019). Survivor guilt in cancer survivorship. *Social Work in Health Care, 58* (8): 764–775.

Goldie, L., & Desmarais, J. (2005). Psychotherapy and the treatment of cancer patients. In: *Treatment of Cancer Patients: Bearing Cancer in Mind.* London: Routledge.

Guardian, The (2003). *Primary School Teaching Resources: The Myth of Pandora's Box.* Available at: https://www.theguardian.com/education/2003/jul/01/primaryschoolteachingresources.primaryeducation

Hall, A. (2003). Trauma and containment in children's cancer treatment. *International Journal of Infant Observation, 6* (2): 111–126.

Hedges, F. (2005). *An Introduction to Systemic Therapy with Individuals: A Social Constructionist Approach.* London: Red Globe Press.

Heidegger, M. (1962). *Being and Time.* Oxford: Blackwell.

Herbert, A., Lyratzopoulos, G., Whelan, J., Taylor, R. M., Barber, J., Gibson, F., & Fern, L. A. (2018). Diagnostic timeliness in adolescents and young adults with cancer: A cross-sectional analysis of the BRIGHTLIGHT cohort. *Lancet Child & Adolescent Health, 2* (3): 180–190.

Hitchens, C. (2012). *Mortality.* London: Atlantic Books.

Holland, J. C. (2018). Psycho-oncology: Overview, obstacles and opportunities. *Psycho-Oncology, 27*: 1364–1376.

Holland, J. C., Breitbart, W. S., Butow, P. N., Jacobsen, P. B., Loscalzo, M. J., & McKorkle, R. (Eds.) (2015). *Psycho-Oncology, Third Edition.* New York: Oxford University Press.

Holland, L., & Thompson, K. (2018). Psychological support and social care. In: J. Chisholm, R. Hough, & L. Soanes (Eds.), *A Practical Approach to the*

Care of Adolescents and Young Adults with Cancer. Cham, Switzerland: Springer.

Hollis, R., & Morgan, S. (2001). The adolescent with cancer—at the edge of no-man's land. *The Lancet Oncology, 2* (1): 43–48.

Janoff-Bulman, R. (1992). *Shattered Assumptions: Towards a New Psychology of Trauma*. New York: Free Press.

Judd, D. (2001). To walk the last bit on my own—narcissistic independence or identification with good objects: Issues of loss for a 13-year-old who had an amputation. *Journal of Child Psychotherapy, 27* (1): 47–67.

Judd, D. (2013). Understanding the patient with cancer. In: J. Burke (Ed.), *The Topic of Cancer: New Perspectives on the Emotional Experience of Cancer*. London: Karnac.

Kazak, A. E., & Noll, R. B. (2015). The integration of psychology in pediatric oncology research and practice: Collaboration to improve care and outcomes for children and families. *American Psychologist, 70* (2): 146–158.

Keegan, T. H. M., Ries, L. A. G., Barr, R. D., & Geiger, A. M. (2016). Comparison of cancer survival trends in the United States of adolescents and young adults with those in children and older adults. *Cancer, 122* (7): 1009–1016.

Kilmer, R. P. (2006). Resilience and posttraumatic growth in children. In: L. G. Calhoun & R. G. Tedeschi (Eds.), *Handbook of Posttraumatic Growth: Research and Practice* (pp. 264–288). New York: Lawrence Erlbaum Associates.

Kissane, D. (2017). Diagnosis and treatment of demoralization. In: M. Watson & D. Kissane (Eds.), *Management of Clinical Depression and Anxiety*. Oxford: Oxford University Press.

Kissane, D. W. (2022). The flourishing scholarship of psychosocial oncology viewed across 30 years through the lens of this journal, Psycho-Oncology. *Psycho-Oncology, 31*: 559–561.

Kitwood, T. (1997). *Dementia Reconsidered: The Person Comes First*. Buckingham: Open University Press.

Klass, D., & Steffen, E. M. (2018). Introduction: Continuing bonds—20 years on. In: D. Klass & E. M. Steffen (Eds.), *Continuing Bonds in Bereavement: New Directions for Research and Practice* (pp. 1–14). New York: Routledge.

Klein, M. (1946a). *Envy and Gratitude*. London: Virago.

Klein, M. (1946b). Notes on some schizoid mechanisms. In: *Envy and Gratitude and Other Works 1946–1963*. London: Vintage, 1997.

Kreicbergs, U., Valdimarsdottir, U., Onelov, E., Henter, J.-I., & Steineck, G. (2004). Talking about death with children who have severe malignant disease. *New England Journal of Medicine, 351* (12): 1175–1186.

Lang, P., & McAdams, E. (1995). Stories, giving accounts and systemic descriptions. Perspectives and positions in conversations. Feeding and fanning the winds of creative imagination. *Human Systems, 6*: 71–103.

Lanyado, M. (1999). Brief psychotherapy and therapeutic consultations: How much therapy is "good-enough"? In: M. Lanyado & A. Horne (Eds.), *The Handbook of Child and Adolescent Psychotherapy*. London: Routledge.

Lee, P. L. (2013). Making now precious: Working with survivors of torture and asylum seekers. *International Journal of Narrative Therapy and Community Work, 1*: 1–10.

Lee, P. L. (2020). *Chatting about the Liminal Space during Covid-19*. Available at: www.narrativeimaginings.com/blog/chatting-about-the-liminal-space-during-covid-19

Lee, T., & Elfer, J. (2013). The emotional impact of cancer on children and their families. In: J. Burke (Ed.), *The Topic of Cancer: New Perspectives on the Emotional Experience of Cancer* (pp. 49–64). London: Karnac.

London Cancer (2014). *Service Specification Psychological Support Services*. Available at: http://londoncancer.org/media/89175/psychological-service-specification-final-2014june-.pdf

Lyratzopoulos, G., Neal, R. D., Barbiere, J. M., Rubin, G. P., & Abel, G. A. (2012). Variation in number of general practitioner consultations before hospital referral for cancer: Findings from the 2010 National Cancer Patient Experience Survey in England. *Lancet Oncology, 13* (4): 353–365.

Macmillan Cancer Support (2013). *Impact Briefs: Psychological and Emotional Support*. Available at: https://www.macmillan.org.uk/_images/Psychological-and-Emotional-Support_tcm9–283186.pdf

Macmillan Cancer Support (2021). *Help with How You're Feeling*. Available at: www.macmillan.org.uk/cancer-information-and-support/get-help/emotional-help

McCabe, M. G. (2018). Overview of adolescent and young adult cancer. In: J. Chisholm, R. Hough, & L. Soanes (Eds.), *A Practical Approach to the Care of Adolescents and Young Adults with Cancer* (pp. 1–18). Cham, Switzerland: Springer.

McCarthy, M. C., McNeil, R., Drew, S., Dunt, D., Kosola, S., & Orme, L. (2016). Psychological distress and posttraumatic stress symptoms in adolescents and young adults with cancer and their parents. *Journal of Adolescent and Young Adult Oncology, 5* (4): 322–329.

McFarland, D., & Holland, J. (2017). Distress, adjustment and anxiety disorders. In: M. Watson & D. Kissane (Eds.), *Management of Clinical Depression and Anxiety*. London: Oxford University Press.

McLeod, J. (1997). *Narrative and Psychotherapy*. London: Sage.

McMonagle, L. M. (2018). Nurse-led ambulatory care. In: P. Olsen & S. Smith (Eds.), *Nursing Adolescents and Young Adults with Cancer*. Cham, Switzerland: Springer.

McParland, J., & Camic, P. M. (2018). How do lesbian and gay people experience dementia? *Dementia, 17*: 452–477.

McParland, J., Khan, I., & Casdagli, L. (2019). Marking our journeys alongside young people. *Clinical Psychology Forum, 320*: 35–37.

Mees, P. (2017). State of mind assessments. *Journal of Child Psychotherapy, 43* (3): 380–394.

Meichenbaum, D. (2012). *Roadmap to Resilience: A Guide for Military, Trauma Victims and Their Families*. Clearwater, FL: Institute Press.

Meltzer, D. (1994). Temperature and distance as technical dimensions of interpretation. In: *Sincerity and Other Works: Collected Papers of Donald Meltzer* (pp. 374–386), ed. A. Hahn. London: Karnac.

Menzies Lyth, I. (1988). *Containing Anxiety in Institutions*. London: Free Association Books.

Mooney, S., Jacobson, C., Chesman, N., & Mann, A. (2016). Promoting wellbeing and resilience. In: S. Smith, S. Mooney, M. Cable, & R. M. Taylor (Eds.), *The Blueprint of Care for Teenagers and Young Adults with Cancer* (2nd edition). London: Teenage Cancer Trust.

Morgan, A. (2000). *What Is Narrative Therapy? An Easy-to-Read Introduction*. Adelaide: Dulwich Centre Publications.

Morgan, S., Davies, S., Palmer, S., & Plaster, M. (2010). Sex, drugs, and rock 'n' roll: Caring for adolescents and young adults with cancer. *Journal of Clinical Oncology, 28* (32): 4825–4830.

Moxley-Haegert, L. (2012). *Hopework*: Stories of Survival from the C.O.U.R.A.G.E Program: Families of Children Diagnosed with cancer*. Available at: https://dulwichcentre.com.au/wp-content/uploads/2014/08/Hopework_by_Linda_Moxley-Haegert.pdf

National Cancer Institute (2001). *Cancer Progress Report*. Bethesda, MD: NIH. Available at: https://www.progressreport.cancer.gov/sites/default/files/archive/report2001.PDF

National Cancer Institute (2022). *Cancer Trends Progress Report*. Bethesda, MD: NIH. Available at: https://www.progressreport.cancer.gov

Naylor, C., Parsonage, M., McDaid, D., Knapp, M., Fossey, M., & Galea, A. (2012). *Long-Term Conditions and Mental Health: The Cost of Co-Morbidities*. London: The Kings Fund & Centre for Mental Health.

NCI (2020). *Dictionary of Cancer Terms*. Available at: www.cancer.gov/publications/dictionaries/cancer-terms/def/late-effect

Ncube, N. (2006). The Tree of Life Project: Using narrative ideas in work with vulnerable children in Southern Africa. *International Journal of Narrative Therapy and Community Work, 1*: 3–16.

NHSE (2013). *Service Specifications: TYA Principal Treatment Centres and Networks*. Available at: https://www.engage.england.nhs.uk/consultation/teenager-and-young-adults-cancer-services/user_uploads/service-specification-tya-principal-treatment-centres-and-networks.pdf

NICE (2005). *Improving Outcomes Guidance for Children and Young People with Cancer*. London: National Institute for Health Care and Clinical Excellence/Crown Publishers.

NICE (2014). *Cancer Services for Children and Young People*. Available at: https://www.nice.org.uk/guidance/qs55/chapter/Quality-statement-4-Psychological-and-social-support

O'Hara, C., Moran, A., Whelan, J. S., & Hough, R. S. (2015). Trends in survival for teenagers and young adults with cancer in the UK 1992–2006. *European Journal of Cancer, 51* (14): 2039–2048.

Patel, N. (2019). Conceptualising rehabilitation as reparation for torture survivors: A clinical perspective. *International Journal of Human Rights, 23*: 1546–1568.

Pena, C., & Garcia, L. (2016). A story of political consciousness and struggle across time and place. In: T. Afuape & G. Hughes (Eds.), *Liberation Practices: Towards Emotional Wellbeing through Dialogue* (pp. 174–184). London: Routledge.

Pennebaker, J. W. (1997). *Opening Up: The Healing Power of Emotional Expression*. New York: Guilford Press.

Perez, S., & Greenzang, K. A. (2019). Completion of adolescent cancer treatment: Excitement, guilt, and anxiety. *Pediatrics, 143* (3): e20183073.

Pitman, A., Suleman, S., Hyde, N., & Hodgkiss, A. (2018). Depression and anxiety in patients with cancer. *British Medical Journal, 361*: k1415.

Polkinghorne, D. E. (1988). *Narrative Knowing and the Human Sciences*. Albany, NY: State University of New York Press.

Portnoy, S., Girling, I., & Fredman, G. (2016). Supporting young people living with cancer to tell their stories in ways that make them stronger: The Beads of Life approach. *Clinical Child Psychology and Psychiatry, 21*: 255–267.

Potamianou, A. (1997). *Hope: A Shield in the Economy of Borderline States*. London: Routledge.

Reder, P., & Fredman, G. (1996). The relationship to help: Interacting beliefs about the treatment process. *Clinical Child Psychology and Psychiatry, 1* (3): 457–467.

Reynolds, V. (2011). Resisting burnout with justice-doing. *International Journal of Narrative Therapy and Community Work, 4*: 27–45.

Reynolds, V. (2012). An ethical stance for justice-doing in community work and therapy. *Journal of Systemic Therapies, 31* (4): 18–33.

Rugbjerg, K., Mellemkjaer, L., & Boice, J. D. (2014). Cardiovascular disease in survivors of adolescent and young adult cancer: A Danish cohort study, 1943–2009. *Journal of the National Cancer Institute, 106* (6): dju110.

Rugbjerg, K., & Olsen, J. H. (2016). Long-term risk of hospitalization for somatic diseases in survivors of adolescent or young adult cancer. *JAMA Oncology, 2* (2): 193–200.

Schulte, F., Brinkman, T., Li, C., Fay-McClymont, T., Srivastava, D. K., Ness, K. K., et al. (2018). Social adjustment in adolescent survivors of pediatric central nervous system tumors: A report from the Childhood Cancer Survivor Study. *Cancer, 124:* 3596–3608.

Seitz, D. C., Besier, T., & Goldbeck, L. (2009). Psychosocial interventions for adolescent cancer patients: A systematic review of the literature. *Psycho-oncology, 18* (7): 683–690.

Servitzoglou, M., Papadatou, D., Tsiantis, I., & Vasilatou-Kosmidis, H. (2008). Psychosocial functioning of young adolescent and adult survivors of childhood cancer. *Supportive Care in Cancer, 16:* 29–36.

Spinelli, E. (1997). *Tales of Un-Knowing: Therapeutic Encounters from an Existential Perspective.* London: Duckworth.

Spinelli, E. (2014). *Practising Existential Psychotherapy: The Relational World* (2nd edition). London: Sage.

Stark, D., Bielack, S., & Brugieres, L. (2016). Teenagers and young adults with cancer in Europe: From national programmes to a European integrated coordinated project. *European Journal of Cancer Care (Engl.), 25* (3): 419–427.

Stark, D., & Ferrari, A. (2018). Models of delivery of care for AYA. In: J. Chisholm, R. Hough, & L. Soanes (Eds.), *A Practical Approach to the Care of Adolescents and Young Adults with Cancer* (pp. 37–55). Cham, Switzerland: Springer.

Steele, A., Mullins, L., Mullins, A. J., & Muriel, A. C. (2015). Psychosocial interventions and therapeutic support as a standard of care in pediatric oncology. *Pediatric Blood Cancer, 62* (5): S585–S618.

Stein, A., Dalton, L., Rapa, E., Bluebond-Langner, M., Hanington, L., Fredman Stein, K., et al. (2019). Communication with children and adolescents about the diagnosis of their own life-threatening condition. *Lancet, 393* (10176): 1150–1163.

Stroebe, M., & Schut, H. (1999). The dual process model of coping with bereavement: Rationale and description. *Death Studies, 23* (3): 197–224.

Tonkin, L. (1996). Growing around grief—another way of looking at grief and recovery. *Bereavement Care, 15* (1): 10.

Tricoli, J. V., Blair, D. G., Anders, C. K., & Bleyer, W. A. (2016). Biologic and clinical characteristics of adolescent and young adult cancers: Acute lymphoblastic leukemia, colorectal cancer, breast cancer, melanoma and sarcoma. *Cancer, 122* (7): 1017–1028.

van der Kolk, B. A. (2014). *The Body Keeps the Score: Brain, Mind, and Body in the Healing of Trauma.* New York: Viking.

Vermeire, S. (2017). What if . . . I were a king?: Playing with roles and positions in narrative conversations with children who have experienced trauma. *International Journal of Narrative Therapy and Community Work, 4:* 50–61.

Vrinten, C., McGregor, M., Heinrich, M., von Wagner, C., Waller, J., Wardle, J., & Black, B. (2017). What do people fear about cancer? A systematic review and meta-synthesis of cancer fears in the general population. *Psycho-Oncology*, 26: 1070–1079.

Waddell, M. (2018). *On Adolescence: Inside Stories*. London: Routledge.

Wade, A. (1997). Small acts of living: Everyday resistance to violence and other forms of oppression. *Contemporary Family Therapy, 19* (1): 23–39.

Walliams, D. (2016). *The Midnight Gang*. London: HarperCollins.

Weingarten, K. (2000). Witnessing, wonder and hope. *Family Process, 39* (4): 389–402.

Weingarten, K. (2010). Reasonable hope: Constructs, clinical applications and support. *Family Process, 49* (1): 5–25.

Weingarten, K. (2012). Sorrow: A therapist's reflection on the inevitable and the unknowable. *Family Process, 51*: 440–455.

White, M. (1995). *Re-Authoring Lives: Interviews and Essays*. Adelaide: Dulwich Centre Publications.

White, M. (1997a). *Narratives of Therapists Lives*. Adelaide: Dulwich Centre Publications.

White, M. (1997b). Challenging the culture of consumption: Rites of passage and communities of acknowledgement. *Dulwich Centre Newsletter, 2* (3): 38–42.

White, M. (1988). *Saying Hullo Again: The Incorporation of the Lost Relationship in the Resolution of Grief*. Adelaide: Dulwich Centre Publications.

White, M. (2007). *Maps of Narrative Practice*. New York: W. W. Norton.

White, M., & Epston, D. (1990). *Narrative Means to Therapeutic Ends*. New York: W. W. Norton.

WHO (2021). *Cancer in Children*. Geneva: World Health Organization.

Wiener, L., Battles, H., Bernstein, D., Long, L., Derdak, J., Mackall, C. L., & Mansky, P. J. (2006), Persistent psychological distress in long-term survivors of paediatric sarcoma: The experience at a single institution. *Psycho-Oncology, 15*: 898–910.

Wiener, L., Kazak, A. E., Noll, R. B., Patenaude, A. F., & Kupst, M. J. (2015). Standards for the psychosocial care of children with cancer and their families: An introduction to the Special Issue. *Pediatric Blood Cancer, 62* (5): S419–S424.

Wiener, L., Pao, M., Kazak, A., Kupst, M., & Patenaude, A. (Eds.) (2014). *Pediatric Psycho-Oncology: A Quick Reference on the Psychosocial Dimensions of Cancer Symptom Management*. London: Oxford University Press.

Winnicott, D. W. (1960). The theory of the parent–infant relationship. *The Maturational Processes and the Facilitating Environment*. London: Karnac, 1990.

Winnicott, D. W. (1961). Struggling through the doldrums. In: *The Family and Individual Development*. London: Tavistock Publications.

Winslade, J. (2002). Storying professional identity: From an interview with John Winslade. *International Journal of Narrative Therapy and Community Work*, 4: 33–38.

Wolf, A. (1991). *Get Out of My Life, but First Could You Drive Me and Cheryl to the Mall? A Parent's Guide to the New Teenager*. New York: Noonday Press.

Worden, J. W. (2009). *Grief Counselling and Grief Therapy: A Handbook for the Mental Health Practitioner*. New York: Springer.

Yalom, I. D. (2002). *The Gift of Therapy: An Open Letter to a New Generation of Therapists and Their Patients*. New York: Harper Collins.

Yalom, I. D. (2017). *Becoming Myself: A Psychiatrist's Memoir*. New York: Basic Books.

Yehuda, N. (2016). *Communicating Trauma: Clinical Presentations and Interventions with Traumatised Children*. London: Routledge.

Yuen, A. (2009). Less pain, more gain: Explorations of responses versus effects when working with the consequences of trauma. *Explorations: An E-Journal of Narrative Practice*, 1: 6–16.

Zebrack, B. J. (2011). Psychological, social, and behavioral issues for young adults with cancer. *Cancer, 117* (10, Suppl.): 2289–2294.

INDEX

Abel, G. A., 8
acknowledgment, communities of, 133
ACP, 14: *see* Association of Child
    Psychotherapists
activity coordinators, 12, 31, 37, 38
adjustment reactions to cancer
    treatment, 10
adolescence:
    cancer in, trauma perspective on,
      79–92
    challenges to authority, conformity,
      and convention in, 8
    definition, 46
    emotional upheaval in, 104
    volatility of, 109
adolescent(s), impact of cancer on, 46–61
adolescents and young adults [AYA], 8
    as "lost tribe" of cancer patients, 7
adolescent ward, measure of disturbance
    on, 47
afterlife, 138
Afuape, T., 127, 129
age-appropriate setting, treatment of
    TYA patients in, 9
Ahmad, S. S., 10
Ajithkumar, T. V., 11
Albritton, K., 7

Aldiss, S., 12, 47
amputations, managing, 90
amygdala, 83
anaesthetists, 37
Anders, C. K., 8
Anderson, B., 7, 30, 141
anhedonia, 30
anhedonic/clinical depression, 39–40
anticipatory anxiety and panic
    attacks, 25
anticipatory nausea, 10, 38
antidepressant, 40, 42
antifungal treatment, 40
anxiety and risks across the team,
    holding: "Dora" (patient
    vignette), 28–29
Association of Child Psychotherapists
    [ACP], 14
assumptive world, shattering of, 80–83
asylum seekers, 126
attention deficit hyperactivity disorder
    [ADHD], 24
authority, conformity, and convention in,
    challenges to, in adolescence and
    young-adulthood, 8
autobiographical memories, 43
AYA: *see* adolescents and young adults

baby:
    impact of invasive medical treatment
        on, 101
    terror of, as nameless dread, 54
Barbiere, J. M., 8
Barnett, M., 11
Barr, R. D., 7, 8, 35
Beads of Life, 5, 131, 133
Becker, E., 85
Behan, C., 77
behavioural experiments, 15
being-in-the-world, 79
    new way of, 86–90
bell, celebratory, 41
Benowitz, S., 8
bereavement, coping processes during,
    136
bereavement support, 47
    charity/"third-sector", 45
    psychological, 44
bereavement theories, 135–137
Berg, I. K., 128
Bergum, V., 5, 126
Bertrando, P., 139
Besier, T., 11
betrayal, sense of, 98
Bick, E., 54, 102
Bielack, S., 8
biographical narrative:
    break in, "Anna" (patient vignette),
        105
    discontinuity in, 94
Bion, W. R., 54, 101
Birch, R., 8
Blair, D. G., 8
blame, projection of, 52
Bleyer, A., 7, 8
Bleyer, W. A., 8
Blomberg, B., 100
blood clots, 39
bodily envelope, breaking of, 49
body image, 55
    disturbances in, 110
Boice, J. D., 8
bone cancer, 22, 26
bone marrow, 93
    transplant, 84, 85
bone or soft-tissue sarcomas, 10
borderline patients, 121
Boscolo, L., 139
Bowlby, J., 80

brain pathology, direct, 10
brain tumour(s), 10, 13, 87, 90, 127
Brennan, J., 80
Brewin, C., 79, 80, 83
Britton, R., 33
Bruce, M., 10
Brugieres, L., 8
Buber, M., 92
Budd, T., 8
Burgess, N., 79
Burnham, J., 128

Caligiuri, M., 7
CAMHS, 28, 53, 124
CAMHS team, 28, 29
Camic, P. M., 125
cancer (passim):
    in adolescence, trauma perspective,
        79–92
    bone, 22, 26
    childhood, 4, 93, 94, 97, 100, 103, 104,
        105, 111
        survivors of, 110
    as existential trauma, 79
    eye, 110
    impact of, on adolescents, 46–61
    "late effects" of, emotional
        complexities arising from
        childhood, 93–111
    perception of:
        as contagious, 96
        as parasite, 95
        as punishment, 95
    relapse of, 41
    as shattering structures of safety and
        certainty: "Mohamed" (patient
        vignette), 3, 81–82
    social consequences of, 11
    stages of treatment, 23, 24
    stigma associated with, 36
    in teenagers and young adults, 7–34
    trauma of, 79
    in young adulthood, services for, 62
cancer diagnosis (passim):
    adjustment reaction following:
        "Shinique" (patient vignette), 38
    co-creating how to live alongside
        cancer: "Olivia" (patient
        vignette), 65–67
    coming to terms with, 37
    experience of, 8

gravity of, awareness of, 63
"Henry" (patient vignette), 51
"Jackie" (patient vignette), 50–51
terminal, 70
and trauma, 3
cancer journey, 23, 75
    commencing treatment, 38–39
    diagnosis, 36–38
    disease progression and palliation,
        44–45
    during treatment, 39–40
    end of treatment, 40–44
    pre-diagnosis, 35–36
    relapse, 44–45
Cancer and Leukaemia in Childhood
    [CLIC], 10, 11, 12
cancer multidisciplinary team [MDT], 10,
    13, 31–34, 38, 53, 61, 142
Cancer Research report on teenage and
    young adult cancer, 9
Cancer Research UK, 8, 9, 10
cancer statistics, 9–10
cancer survival rates, 8
cancer treatment (passim):
    adjustment reactions to, 10
    end of, 3, 40, 41, 56, 58, 81, 82, 90
    experience of, 8
    familiarity with: "Damian" (patient
        vignette), 24–25
    flashbacks and nightmares after end
        of: "Jonny" (patient vignette),
        83–87
    "here-and-now" frustrations of, 23
    impact of, 3
    in infancy, 94
    intravenous, 9
    isolation from friends during:
        "Harold" (patient vignette), 55
    "late effects" of, 3, 29, 43, 115
    need to change clinicians, approach,
        and teams in: "Clem" (patient
        vignette), 21–22
    outcomes, 8
    phobia of components of, 10
    in pre-verbal period, 94
    psychological support in, 10–12
    radio-isotope, 24
    resulting in mistrust of people:
        "Verity" (patient vignette), 4,
        108–109
    toll of, 30

cancer treatment model, aligning
    symptoms to: "Penny" (patient
    vignette), 25
Carbone, P., 95
car crash, 80
cardiologists, 37
Cardona, L., 10
Carr, R., 9
Carter, C., 63
Casdagli, L., 133
causes, search for, 94–97
    "Chloe" (patient vignette), 95–97
    "Kieron" (patient vignette), 96
    parents': "Mr and Ms Oyekan"
        (patient vignette), 96
CBT: see cognitive behavioural therapy
CCLG: see Children's Cancer and
    Leukaemia Group
Cecchin, G., 91
celebratory bell, 41
central nervous system (brain and spinal
    cord) tumours, 8
central nervous system
    inflammation, 10
chemotherapy (passim):
    emotional repercussions of, 29
    late effects of, 93
    panic attacks preceding, 38
    side-effects of, 10, 17, 18
Chesman, N., 10
child(ren) (passim):
    with early physical experiences of
        pain, 100
    life-limiting disease of, parents'
        anguish in face of: "Tessa"
        (patient vignette), 119
    loss of, 6, 142
childhood, early, trauma in, 100–102
childhood cancer (passim):
    adult survivor of, 111
    impact on family of, 111
    survivors of, 110
Children, Teenage and Young Adult
    Psych-Oncology Team, 13
chronic fatigue, 90
chronic health conditions, 98, 125
chronic sorrow, 6, 132
CLIC: see Cancer and Leukaemia in
    Childhood
CLIC Sargent, 10, 11, 12
clinical/anhedonic depression, 39–40

clinical nurse specialists [CNS],
    oncology, 12
cognitive behavioural therapy [CBT], 14,
    15, 25
cognitive changes, 90
cognitive functioning, impact on, 94
cognitive neuroscience, 79
collective sustainability, 142
Colloms, A., 100
communities of acknowledgment,
    133
Community Paediatric Palliative Care
    Team, Life Force, 123
compassion, integrative approaches
    drawing on, 79
Connexions workers, 31
containment, 134
    psychoanalytic theory of, 101
    role of skin in, 102
continuity-of-being, 104
continuity of life and development,
    break in: "Hasina" (patient
    vignette), 103
Cooke, M., 8
Cooper, M., 92
countertransference, definition, 14
COVID-19 pandemic, 19, 31, 90
cranio-spinal radiation treatment, 13
curiosity, therapeutic stance of, 91

Dalal, C., 91
Damaskos, P., 41
Datta, S. S., 10, 11, 16
Davies, A., 110
Davies, S., 8
death:
    of adolescent, 58–61
    of child, 6, 142
    child facing, 134
    and dying, talking with young people
        about, 70–77
    facing, 123, 124, 125, 134
    fear of, 27, 70, 78, 80
        imminent, re-connecting: "Priya"
        (patient vignette), 75–77
    of patient: "Aydin" (patient
        vignette), 60
    talking about, 65, 76
    untameability of, 6, 143
    work with people facing, role of
        psychology in, 125–127

young person facing, working with
    families of, 123–143
decentred and influential position, of
    therapists, 129
Dein, S., 96
dementia, 125, 134
demoralization vs anhedonic/clinical
    depression, 39–40
Denborough, D., 126
denial, 32, 36, 37, 74, 77
    as kind of knowing, 138
depression, 10, 39, 40, 53, 110
    reactive, 115
De Shazer, S., 128
Desmarais, J., 102
despair, in face of life-threatening
    disease, 112–122
developmental milestones, young
    people's, ability to reach, 9
diagnosis of cancer, see cancer diagnosis
diarrhoea, 108
dieticians, 31, 37
disability, 103
disease:
    incurable, 70
    life-threatening, 52, 112
disfigurement, 103
disseminated fungal infection, 40
dissociating, definition, 21
documentation, 127
Dommett, R. M., 35
Dossetor, J., 5, 126
double-storied accounts, 131
drug misuse, 110
dual process model, 136
Dye, K. P., 110

Edwards, M., 9
Eilertsen, M.-E. B., 110
Elfer, J., 1–16, 46, 101
Emanuel, R., 100
embodiment, 126
EMDR: see eye movement
        desensitisation and reprocessing
        therapy
emotional memories, resurfacing of, 43
emotional self, centring, 130
employment, 8, 31
    issues around, in young adulthood, 62
endocrinologists, 37
engagement, 19, 64, 126

environment, 100, 101, 106, 126
Epston, D., 87
existential phenomenology, 81, 83, 91
existential trauma, 82
    cancer as, 79
explosion of *noema*, 80
eye movement desensitisation and
        reprocessing [EMDR] therapy, 3,
        79, 83, 84, 85

family(ies):
    re-enactment of problems in, within
        the MDT: "Pete" (patient
        vignette), 33–34
    of young person facing death, working
        with, 123–143
Fann, J., 12
fatalistic thinking, 129
father, feelings of guilt of: "Mr Arden"
        (patient vignette), 97
fatigue, chronic, 90
fear, projection of, 52
Fearon, P., 10
Feltbower, R. G., 110
Fern, L. A., 8
Ferrari, A., 8, 9, 13, 31, 36
fertility, 5, 37, 95, 98, 103
    issues around, in young adulthood, 62
    issues with, 90
Fidler, M., 110
financial issues, 97
first contact:
    reflections from, importance of,
        19–20
    with young person, radical importance
        of, 20
Fisher, J., 79
flashbacks, 80, 83, 84, 85
flashbacks and nightmares, after end
        of treatment: "Jonny" (patient
        vignette), 83–87
float-back, 84
Flynn, D., 46, 47
fractured memory, 83
Fredman, G., 5, 16, 64, 72, 75, 91, 129, 130,
        131, 138, 140, 142
Freud, A., 109
Freud, S., 101
Friend, A. J., 110
further education, issues around, in
        young adulthood, 62

fury, projection of, 52
future, sense of loss about: "Kate"
        (patient vignette), 120

Galloway, A., 2, 5, 62–78
Garcia, L., 132
Garland, C., 49
gastroenterologists, 37
Geiger, A. M., 8
Geiger counter, 24
genitals, cancer of, 50
Girling, I., 5, 131
Glaser, A. W., 110
Glaser, S., 41
Glazer, D., 3, 79–92
Goldbeck, L., 11
Goldie, L., 102
Goolishian, H., 141
Greenzang, K. A., 41
Gregory, J., 79
grief, growing around, 136
Groszmann, M., 1, 7, 35–73
growth:
    effect on, 103
    reduced, 93, 109
guilt, 94
    feelings of, 97–100
        father's: "Mr Arden" (patient
            vignette), 97
        for having cancer: "Chloe" (patient
            vignette), 97
        mother's: "Baby Tamsin" (patient
            vignette), 98
        mother's: "Ms Rodriguez" (patient
            vignette), 99
        survivor: "Anna" (patient vignette),
            105
        survivor: "Keith" (patient
            vignette), 98
Gumley, D., 10

haematological malignancy(ies), 8, 9, 28
haematologists, 31
hair:
    bodily, loss of, 69
    loss of, 18, 51, 55, 58, 101, 109
    fear of, 50, 108
Hall, A., 102, 107, 108
Hamilton, W., 35
Hatcher, H. M., 11
health psychology, 14

heart problems, risk of, 94
Hedges, F., 64, 66
Heidegger, M., 79, 89, 90
helplessness, feelings of, 18, 33, 99, 101, 109
Henry, C., 4, 5, 112–122
Henter, J.-I., 59
Herbert, A., 46, 48
high-grade glioma brain-tumours, 9–10
hippocampus, 83
historical narrative, gaps in, 106
Hitchens, C., 52
Hodgkin's lymphoma, 17, 91
Hodgkiss, A., 11
Holland, J., 10, 11
Holland, L., 10, 11, 16
Hollis, R., 7, 9
hope:
    holding on to, 6, 128
    in face of life-threatening disease, 112–122
    projection of, 52
    reasonable, 6, 128
    unrealistic, as "defensive shield in borderline cases", 120
Hope, Pandora's dragonfly, 4, 112, 113, 115
Hopework, 131
hospital schools, 9
Hough, R. S., 8
Hughes, E. J., 110
humanistic belief, 139
Husserl, E., 3, 80
Hyde, N., 11

identity:
    development of, 94
    liminal space for, 132
    migration of, 132, 133
    preferred, 69, 75, 90, 134
    reclaiming and cancer-free: "Josh" (patient vignette), 67–69
illness, relational nature of, 2, 62–63
incontinence, 18
indestructibility, feeling of, and search for excitement: "Deepak" (patient vignette), 109
Indredavik, M. S., 110
infancy:
    cancer in, 4
    trauma in, 100–102

infection(s), 30, 39, 56
    disseminated fungal, 40
infectious diseases physicians, 37
infertility, 107
    risk of, 94
integrated self, sense of, development of, 104
internal working models, concept of, 80
interpretations and metaphor, explicit use of: "Adi" (patient vignette), 26
intravenous treatments, 9
intrusive thoughts, 110
invasive medical treatment, impact of, on baby, 101
invasive procedures, 107, 108
Isham, L., 10
I-Thou relationship, 92

Jacobson, C., 10
James Lind Alliance Research Priority Setting Programme, 12
Janoff-Bulman, R., 80
jaundice, 40
Judaism, 140
Judd, D., 56, 96

Kazak, A. E., 10, 11, 38
Keegan, T. H. M., 8
Khan, I., 105, 133
kidney failure, 40
Kilmer, R. P., 90
Kintsugi, Japanese art of, 3, 89
Kissane, D., 10, 11, 39, 40
Kitwood, T., 134
Klass, D., 136
Klein, M., 51
Knowles, K., 41
Kreicbergs, U., 59
Kupst, M., 10, 11

Lang, P., 64
Lanyado, M., 59
late effects, 11, 23
    of cancer treatment, 3, 10, 29, 43, 115
    definition, 10
    emotional complexities arising from childhood cancer, 93–111
    physical and mental, 102
Late Effects Clinic, 21, 93, 106, 107, 111
"Late Effects" Services, 90

Lax-Pericall, M. T., 10
Lee, P. L., 126, 132, 133, 137
Lee, T., 101
lesbian, gay, and bisexual [LGB] people, with dementia, 125
leukaemia, 38, 55, 81, 83, 95, 97, 100
"Level 1–2" psychological support, 11
LGB: see lesbian, gay, and bisexual
liberation psychology, 125
libido, loss of, 30
life:
    or death, issues of, 82
    past, disconnection from: "Keith" (patient vignette), 106
Life Force, 124, 130, 137, 142
    Community Paediatric Palliative Care Team, 123
    Palliative Care Team, 125
life-limiting condition, 139
life-threatening disease, hope and despair in face of, 112–122
limb, loss of, 57
liminal space, 5, 133, 137
    for identity, 132
Lipton, M., 79
living death, 134
Local Authority care, 33
London Cancer, 10
loss:
    accepting reality of, 135
    sense of, 59, 77, 120, 121, 129
    sense of, about future: "Kate" (patient vignette), 120
"lost tribe" of cancer patients, adolescents and young adults as, 7
Lyratzopoulos, G., 8

Macmillan Cancer Support, 10, 11, 12, 13
Macmillan standards, 13
Maggie's, 11
Mahanta, P., 10
making now precious, 137, 138, 141
Mann, A., 10
Martin, R. M., 36
masturbation, 50
maturity, psychological, 90
McAdams, E., 64
McCabe, M. G., 7, 8, 10, 35, 36
McCarthy, M. C., 10
McFarland, D., 10

McGoldrick, M., 63
McLeod, J., 87
McMonagle, L. M., 9
McParland, J., 5, 123–143
MDT: see multidisciplinary team
meaning(s):
    centrality of, to trauma, 83–85
    meaninglessness of, 86
meaninglessness, 82, 86
    role of, 85
measure of disturbance, on adolescent ward, 47
medical complications, demoralization in face of: "Sabina" (patient vignette), 40
medical treatment, invasive, 101
Mees, P., 14
Mehta, S., 111
Meichenbaum, D., 86
Mellemkjaer, L., 8
Meltzer, D., 5, 118
memory(ies):
    autobiographical, 43
    emotional, resurfacing of, 43
    fractured, 83
Memory Day, 136
memories, fear of losing: "Chloe" (patient vignette), 103
Mendelsohn, A., 100
Mental Health Act, 18
Menzies Lyth, I, 116
microbiologists/infectious diseases physicians, 37
migration of identity, 132, 133
mindfulness exercises, 31
mindfulness practices, 15
Mohr, P. A. M., 3, 4, 93–111
Montello, M., 8
Mooney, S., 10, 11, 12
Moran, A., 8
Morgan, A., 135
Morgan, S., 7, 8, 9
mortality (passim):
    awareness of, 91
    confrontation with, 2, 63, 70, 82
    facing, 23, 24, 63, 70, 79, 91, 113
        and not facing, 27
        and not facing: "Bill" (patient vignette), 27–28
    issues of, 85
    making sense of, 80

recognition of, 70
thinking about, 114, 115
mortality rates for cancers, 9
higher proportional, of young
adults, 62
mother:
feeling of break of, in her own life:
"Ms Kahn" (patient vignette),
105–106
feelings of guilt of:
"Baby Tamsin" (patient vignette), 98
and daughter, hope and despair
of: "Amelia" (patient vignette),
116–118
"Ms Rodriguez" (patient
vignette), 99
mothering, good-enough, 100
motivational interviewing, 14
Moxley-Haegert, L., 131
Muller, H., 100
Mullins, A. J., 10
Mullins, L., 10
multidisciplinary psycho-oncology
approach, 14
multidisciplinary risk management, 28
multidisciplinary team [MDT], 10, 53,
70, 142
conscious and unconscious processes
within, 31
meetings, psychosocial, 13
oncology, 13, 31, 34, 38
well-functioning, holistic, 11
Muriel, A. C., 10
Muslim faith, 140

nameless dread, baby's terror as, 54
narrative, break in continuity of, 102–107
"Deepak" (patient vignette), 104
"Hasina" (patient vignette), 103
mother's sense of: "Baby Tamsin"
(patient vignette), 105
narrative therapy, 14, 63, 127, 131, 136
National Cancer Institute [NCI], 8, 10
National Health Service England
[NHSE], 62
National Institute of Health and Care
Excellence [NICE], 7, 9–13
National Institutes of Health [NIH], 10
nausea, 33, 101, 108
anticipatory and conditioned, 10, 38
Naylor, C., 12

NCI [National Cancer Institute], 8, 10
Ncube, N., 130
Neal, R. D., 8
needles, 4, 10, 108, 109
anticipatory anxiety and panic attacks
prior to interventions or tests
with, 25
phobia of, 25, 38
terror of, 25
"Nessun Dorma", 119
neurobiology, of trauma, 83
neuroscience, 3
NHSE [National Health Service
England], 13, 62
NICE [National Institute of Health and
Care Excellence], 7, 9–13
Nichols, C., 7
nightmares, 42, 83, 84, 85
NIH: see National Institutes of Health
noema, 3, 82
definition, 80
explosion of, 80
Noll, R. B., 10, 38
normal life:
dislocation from, 102
return to:
"Margaret" (patient vignette), 57
"Nathan" (patient vignette), 58

occupational therapist(s) [OT], 12, 31, 37,
48, 53
O'Hara, C., 8
Olsen, J. H., 8
"omnipotence", therapeutic, 32
oncologists, consultant, 31
oncology clinical nurse specialists, 12
oncology multidisciplinary team, 13,
34, 38
oncology nurses, 37
Onelov, E., 59
oral steroids, 39
orthopaedic surgeons, 37
OT: see occupational therapist

paediatric cancer services, 106
paediatric haematology, 107
paediatric oncology, 107
paediatric palliative care team, 124
pain, childhood physical experiences of,
100
palliative care, 12, 37, 124, 142

palliative care teams, 12, 37
Palmer, S., 8
Pandora's Box, 4, 112–113, 122
Pao, M., 11
Papadatou, D., 110
paradoxes, 94, 107–110, 111
paralysis, 87
parent(s):
fear of effect on: "Chloe" (patient
vignette), 4
searching for causes: "Mr and Ms
Oyekan" (patient vignette), 96
working through: "Jen" (patient
vignette), 17–18
Patel, N., 135
Patenaude, A., 10, 11
patient vignettes:
"Adi": explicit use of interpretations
and metaphor, 26
"Amber": weakened image of self,
87–89
"Amelia": 121
"Anna":
break in biographical narrative, 105
survivor's guilt, 2, 62, 99, 105, 120
"Annabelle": right time to work on
trauma after cancer, 42–43
"Aydin": death of patient, 60
"Baby Tamsin":
mother's feelings of guilt, 98
mother's sense of break in
continuity of child's narrative, 105
"Bill": holding formulation and
interpretations in mind; facing
and not facing mortality, 27–28
"Chloe":
break in continuity of life and
development and fear of loss of
memories, 103–104
fear of effect on parents, 4
fear of losing memories, 103
feeling guilt for having cancer, 97
question of "why me?", 95–97
"Clem": need to change clinicians,
approach, and teams in treatment,
21, 22
"Damian": familiarity with cancer
treatments, 24, 25
"Deepak":
break in continuity of life and
development, 104

feeling of indestructibility and
search for excitement, 109
"Dora": holding anxiety and risks
across the team, 28, 29
"Harold": isolation from friends
during treatment, 55
"Hasina": break in continuity of life
and development, 103
"Henry": cancer diagnosis, 51
"Jackie": cancer diagnosis, 50–51
"Jen": working through a parent,
17–18
"Jonny": flashbacks and nightmares
after end of treatment, 83–87
"Josh": cancer-free: reclaiming identity,
67–69
"Kate": sense of loss about future, 120
"Keith":
disconnection from past life, 106
survivor guilt, 98
"Kieron":
searching for causes, 96
survivor's feeling of emptiness, 110
"Kiran": working through staff, 18, 19
"Kunle": enabling individual therapy
through parent therapy, 17
"Lyra": speaking about the
unspeakable when cure is not
possible, 71–75
"Margaret": return to "normal life, 57
"Mohamed": cancer as shattering
structures of safety and certainty,
3, 81–82
"Mr Arden": father's feelings of
guilt, 97
"Mr and Ms Oyekan": parents'
searching for causes, 96
"Ms Kahn": mother's feeling of break
in her own life, 105–106
"Ms Rodriguez": mother's feelings of
guilt, 99
"Nathan": return to "normal life", 58
"Olivia": diagnosis: co-creating how to
live alongside cancer, 65–67
"Penny": aligning symptoms to
treatment-model, 25
"Pete": re-enactment of problems
in a family within the MDT,
33, 34
"Pria": process of finding the right
therapist and approach, 22, 23

"Priya": re-connecting when death is imminent, 75–77
"Rachel": first experience of (not) talking, 70–71
"Sabina": demoralization in the face of medical complications, 40
"Shinique": adjustment reaction following diagnosis, 38
"Tessa": parents' anguish in face of child's life-limiting disease, 119
"Verity":
    follow-up visit resulting in self-harm, 4, 108, 109
    treatment resulting in mistrust of people, 4, 108, 109
"Yusuf": Psych-Oncology in role of "interpreter", 39
peer trainers, 133
Pena, C., 5, 6, 123–143
Pennebaker, J. W., 138
people facing death, work with, role of psychology in, 125–127
Perez, S., 41
personality disorder, 22
personhood, 134, 135
pharmacists, 37
phenomenology, 80
    existential, 81, 83, 91
phobias, 38
physiotherapists, 12, 18, 31, 37, 48
physiotherapy, 26
Pitman, A., 11
Plaster, M., 8
play specialist(s), 12, 24, 25, 31, 37, 38, 48
poetic speech, 77
Polkinghorne, D. E., 87
polyphony, 123
Portnoy, S., 5, 123–143
post-chemotherapy phase, 108
post-traumatic growth, 3, 58, 90–91, 142
post-traumatic shock, 3
post-traumatic states of mind, 113
post-traumatic stress, 113
post-traumatic stress disorder [PTSD], 10, 21, 80, 110, 135
Potamianou, A., 120
powerlessness, feelings of, 96, 100, 109
pre-bereavement, 129
preferred identity, 69, 75, 90, 134
pregnancy, issues around, in young adulthood, 62

pre-verbal period, cancer treatment in, 94
primitive fears, 103
primitive splitting, psychoanalytic concept of, 47
process of becoming, self experienced as, 87
projection:
    of blame, 52
    of hope, trust, fury, or fear, 52
    psychoanalytic concept of, 47, 51
projective identification, psychoanalytic concept of, 47, 51
protection racket, 138, 139
protective shell, 80
protective shield, pierced by trauma, 101
psychic skin, of caregiver's containing function, 102
psychodynamic formulations and interpretations, 15
psychodynamic perspectives, 31
psychodynamic psychotherapy(ies), 15, 29
psychodynamic State of Mind assessment, 14
psychological bereavement support, 44
psychological maturity, 90
psychological support (passim):
    in cancer treatment, 10–12
    level of, 11
psychology, role of, in work with people facing death, 125–127
Psych-Oncology Team (passim):
    evolution of, 13–14
    flexible working in, 29–34
    holding anxiety and risk within, 28–29
    multidisciplinary nature of, 22
    processes, 16–34
    referrals to, 1, 12, 13, 16, 31, 42, 64, 83, 103
    in role of "interpreter": "Yusuf" (patient vignette), 39
psycho-oncology, 7–34, 37, 40, 62, 64
    knowledge, experience, and approach in, 23–28
    teenage and young adult, 23
psycho-oncology approach, multidisciplinary, 14
psycho-oncology professionals, 11
psychosocial multidisciplinary team meetings, 13
psychosocial oncology, 11

PTSD: *see* post-traumatic stress disorder
pubertal changes, 109
public health restraining order, 24
punishment, perception of cancer as, 95

radio-isotope treatment, 24
radiologists, 37
radiotherapists, 37
radiotherapy, 26, 41, 53, 93, 98, 107
Rannestad, T., 110
Rapaport, P., 64
reasonable hope, 6, 128
Redaniel, M. T., 35
Reder, P., 16, 64
referrals to Psych-Oncology Team, 1, 12,
      13, 16, 31, 42, 64, 83, 103
refugees, torture rehabilitation centre
      for, 124
reincorporation, 133, 134
Reinius, M. A. V., 10
relational ethics, four key themes of, 126
relational reflexivity, 128
"relationship to help" semi-structured
      interview, 16
religious faith, working with clients with,
      139–141
re-membering conversations, 74, 136
respect, mutual, 5, 126
respectful curiosity, 141
respirator, as monster, 101
Reynolds, V., 126, 141, 142
Ries, L., 8
rites of passage, 133
   ability to experience, 9
Rubin, G. P., 8
Rugbjerg, K., 8

safe place to stand, concept of, 130
sarcomas, 8
   bone or soft-tissue, 10
scars, 57, 109
Schulte, F., 11
Schut, H., 136
second skin, definition, 54
Seitz, D. C., 11
self, experienced as process of becoming,
      weakened image of: "Amber"
      (patient vignette), 87–89
self-care, 6, 142
self-esteem, low, 110
self-harm, 4, 109

self-narrative, disruption to, 132
sensory-motor systems, integrative
      approaches drawing on, 79
Servitzoglou, M., 110, 111
setting, age-appropriate, treatment of
      TYA patients in, 9
sex, unprotected, 2
Sexton, J., 12
Shamanic belief, 121
side-effects, young people's
      physiological sensitivity to, 8
social workers, 31
soft-tissue tumour, 18
solution-focused practice, 128
somatic bridge, 84
somatic complaints, 110
sorrow, chronic, 6, 132
Specialist Commissioning of Cancer
      Services, NHS-England, TYA
      Cancer Primary Treatment
      Centres in, 9
speech and language therapists, 31
Spinelli, E., 81, 85, 88, 91
spirituality, 130, 141
splitting, primitive, psychoanalytic
      concept of, 47
staff, working through: "Kiran" (patient
      vignette), 18–19
staff group, support for, 121
staffing shortages, 31
staff work discussion group, 121
Stark, D., 8, 9, 13, 31, 36
State of Mind assessment,
      psychodynamic, 14
Steele, A., 10
Steffen, E. M., 136
Stein, A., 58, 59
Steineck, G., 59
steroids, 17, 101
   oral, 39
Stevens, M. C. G., 35
stress, traumatic, 10
Stroebe, M., 136
suicidal thoughts, 22, 140
suicide attempt, 28
Suleman, S., 11
superstition, 3
surgeons, orthopaedic, 37
surgery, 26, 68, 69, 98, 101, 109, 114
surveillance appointment,
      42, 43

survival, 8, 9, 36, 43, 98, 99, 103, 104, 110, 116, 126
  struggle for, 100
survivor(s):
  feeling of emptiness of: "Kieron" (patient vignette), 110
  guilt of, 41
    "Anna" (patient vignette), 99
    "Keith" (patient vignette), 98
survivorship care, 47
Sutton, S., 8
symptom control/palliative care teams, 37
systemic family therapy, 14, 29
systemic psychotherapies, 15
systemic thinking, 31

talking, creating space for, 64–70
  first experience of: "Rachel" (patient vignette), 70–71
talking about talking, 72, 129
tattoos, 109
  as self-harm, 4
teenage and young adult [TYA], 2, 8, 12, 64
  cancer, 1, 7–34
    clinical nurse specialist [CNS], 11
    innovations, 9
    patients, 9, 10
  cancer patients, survival rates of, 9
  Cancer Primary Treatment Centres, 9
  in Specialist Commissioning of Cancer Services, NHS-England, 9
  patients, treatment of, in age-appropriate setting, 9
  psychological medicine service, 1
  rites of passage, ability to experience, 9
teenage and young adult [TYA] cancer clinical nurse specialist [CNS], 11, 37, 55, 71, 75
temperature, modulation of, 119
temperature and distance, modulation of, in clinical relationship, 118
terminal diagnosis, 70
terminal illness:
  facing, 44
  talking about, 65
Testa, R., 100
therapeutic documents, 127
therapeutic space, 14

therapist(s):
  and approach, right, process of finding: "Pria" (patient vignette), 22–23
  decentred and influential position of, 129
therapy, parent, enabling individual therapy through: "Kunle" (patient vignette), 17
Thompson, K., 11
thought diaries, 15
Tonkin, L., 136
torture rehabilitation centre for refugees, 124
transference, definition, 14
transplant rejection, 56
trauma:
  of cancer, 79
  centrality of meaning to, 83–85
  etymology of term, 49
  existential, 79, 82
  as experience beyond words, 86
  experience of, 114
  external, 107
  in infancy and early childhood, 100–102
  internal, 107
  neurobiology of, 83
  piercing protective shield, 101
  post-cancer, right time to work on: "Annabelle" (patient vignette), 42–43
  therapeutic approaches focused on, 79
  working in, 122
  young people in grip of, 113
trauma-focused therapy, 21, 83
trauma perspective, on cancer in adolescence, 79–92
trauma therapy(ies), 79, 86
traumatic states of mind, 113, 118
traumatic stress, 10
Tricoli, J. V., 8
trust, projection of, 52
Tsiantis, I., 110
tumour(s), 50, 75
  brain, 87, 90, 127
  central nervous system (brain and spinal cord), 8
  soft-tissue, 18
TYA: *see* teenage and young adult

UK BRIGHTLIGHT study, 46
University College Hospital, 123
University College London Hospital, 91
unknowing, therapeutic stance of, 91
unrealistic hope, as "defensive shield in
    borderline cases", 120
unspeakable, speaking about, when cure
    is not possible: "Lyra" (patient
    vignette), 71–75
urologists/renal physicians, 37

Valdimarsdottir, U., 59
van der Kolk, B. A., 79, 86
Vasilatou-Kosmidis, H., 110
Vermeire, S., 123
Vik, T., 110
vomiting, 108
    anticipatory, 38
Vrinten, C., 95

Waddell, M., 50, 104
Wade, A., 69
Walliams, D., 120
    The Midnight Gang, 119
Webb, A., 111
Weingarten, K., 127, 128, 131, 132, 138
Whelan, J., 8
White, M., 63, 74, 87, 129–133, 135, 136
Whiteson, M., 9

WHO: see World Health Organization
Wiener, L., 10, 11, 110
wig(s), 31, 51, 55
Winnicott, D. W., 48, 104
Winslade, J., 135
withdrawal, 18, 37, 110
Wolf, A., 63
Worden, J. W., 135
World Health Organization [WHO], 9

Yalom, I. D., 80, 83, 91, 92
Yehuda, N., 101
young adults with cancer:
    connectedness of, importance of, 62–78
    services for, 62
young child, with cancer, 4
Young Lives vs Cancer, 11, 31, 37
Young Lives vs Cancer social worker(s),
    11, 12
young person:
    death of, 5
    facing death, working with families of,
        123–143
    first contact with, radical importance
        of, 20
Younus, S., 10
Yuen, A., 142

Zebrack, B. J., 8

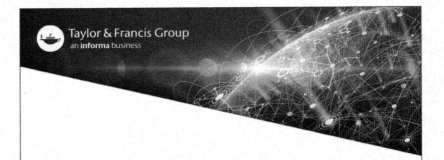